Praise for *Cancer for Two*

"This well-written, organized book is packed with useful information, but it is the special brand of sensitive humor throughout that makes [it] a fascinating, heartwarming treasure. If you want to know how to best care for someone you love so that they can heal and bolster both of your lives with optimism and humor, while preserving your own health, too, then this is one book you must read."
~ Linda Hart, Ph.D., host of "The Hart of It" on HealthyLife.net

"I can't thank you enough for this book. Not only is it completely full of courage, it has completely helped my 'freaked-out' husband to stop dead in his tracks and come back to see that he needs and wants, most of all, to be there right at my side."
~ Gwynith Brennan, Cancer Patient

"Your book has really helped me and let me know what I am feeling is not weird. I really enjoyed your book. Thank you for letting me know I am normal."
~ Denise Dangler, Caregiver

"I am going thru chemo treatments now. I downloaded [Cancer for Two] *so both my husband and I could read it at the same time. I couldn't wait for the book to arrive in the mail so I read the entire download the first day. I loved it! Thanks so much for your wonderful book."*
~ Jody Taylor, Cancer Patient

"[Cancer for Two] *is factual and current and closely relates to what we are going through right now. We were looking for hope and encouragement, along with facts; we found all that and more. One thing Dave said that I have adopted myself... 'don't go there, till you get there'...very profound!! I take it with me everywhere!"*
~ Jo Epperson, Cancer Patient

"...what you have done is create an immediate and complete 'support group' in a book. If I were an oncologist, I would make sure all my patients had it. The book is fantastic: it needs to be out there!"
~ Robert Kotler, MD, FACS
Clinical Instructor, UCLA
Author, *Secrets of a Beverly Hills Cosmetic Surgeon*

"Cancer is more curable with a caregiver that's a love-giver support system. Here's the glorious 'how-to'"
~ Mark Victor Hansen and Jack Canfield,
Co-authors, *Chicken Soup for the Survivor's Soul*

"Honest, funny, and touching, Cancer for Two *will inspire you with Dave and Chris's attitude and courage. Walk with them through that cancer door and find... hope."*
~ Gregory J.P. Godek, Author, *1001 Ways to be Romantic*

"You've found a way to put heart and humor into braving the cancer diagnosis and recovery. It's not sugarcoated – it's the real deal."
~ Judith Parker Harris
Author, *Conquer Crisis with Health-Esteem*

"I wept and I wept harder and cried softly, then of course became sick with hysterical laughter... what a gift! ...whenever I don't feel right or [the doctor] says I'm dropping weight again, I'll just tuck your book of courage under my arm and stand tall and smiling."
~ Lynnda Nafzgar, Cancer Survivor

"I was very moved by your words and what you and Chris have endured. It was a very emotional book for me... lots of crying and laughing, too! Thank you for the experience!"
~ Julie Oaks, Dental Hygienist

"It is awesome and inspiring and will shine a bright light for so many. You have turned something so difficult to face and fight into something of great courage and dignity. Well done!"
~ Kendall S. Wagner, MD
Orthopedic Surgeon

CANCER *for* TWO

An Inspiring True Story and Guide for Cancer Patients and Their Partners

You can handle it.

Dave Balch

Dave Balch

Third edition, revised

A FEW GOOD PEOPLE PAPERBACK

Published by: A Few Good People, Inc.
P.O. Box 824
Twin Peaks, CA 92391

www.CancerForTwo.com

First Printing: 2003
First Revised Edition: 2004
Second Revised Edition: 2006

This book may be purchased in bulk for educational, business, or promotional uses. For information contact: orders@CancerForTwo.com

DISCLAIMER: this book is not intended to replace the services of trained health care or mental health care or social service professionals. The book does not constitute the practice of any medical or other professional health care advice, diagnosis or treatment. Although the author and publisher have made a conscientious effort to provide high quality information, no book can substitute for professional care and advice. You are advised to consult with your personal physician or other professional if you have any healthcare related questions. Accordingly, the author and publisher expressly disclaim any liability, loss, damage, or injury caused by information contained in this book or companion websites.

Publisher's Cataloging-in-Publication

    Balch, Dave.
       Cancer for two / Dave Balch. -- 3rd ed., rev.
       p. cm.
       Includes index.
       ISBN 0-9726901-2-3
       ISBN 0-9726901-1-5

       1. Balch, Chris--Health. 2. Balch, Dave. 3. Breast --Cancer--Popular works. 4. Breast--Cancer--Patients-- Family relationships. 5. Breast--Cancer--Psychological aspects. 6. Caregivers--Family relationships.
       I. Title.

    RC280.B8B353 2006   616.99'449'00922
                        QBI06-200070

For Christine:
you have earned a Purple Heart for bravery,
and my heart for life.

*"To love someone deeply gives you strength.
Being loved by someone deeply gives you courage."*
Lao Tzu

Table of Contents

About the Author.. xi
Acknowledgements.. xiii
Introduction..17
   Internet Extras and Services.......................................22

April 10: The Lump and Biopsy..23
April 22: The Diagnosis..26
Giving Permission 41
April 24: The Surgeon 45
Dealing with People...48
April 29: The First Second Opinion....................................58
May 1: The New York Book Expo 66
May 10: The Lumpectomy and Sentinel Node Biopsy........70
May 15: The Post Op Appointment.....................................83
May 17: The Second Second Opinion..................................88
May 19: The Star Wars Incident...94
Pac-Man..97
May 20: The Bone Scan..99
The Big Decision 101
June 3: UCLA at Night..106
June 10: The Pre-op, School, and Eclipse.......................110
June 12: The Multi-Disciplinary Conference 119
June 13: Mastectomy and Reconstruction.......................126
June 17: Coming Home 141
June 24: The Post-Op Appointment..................................153
June 25: The Midnight Ride..155
July 9: The Chemotherapy Consult 163
July 12: 1st Chemotherapy Treatment 168
August 1: 2nd Chemotherapy Treatment...........................176
August 23: 3rd Chemotherapy Treatment..........................183
September 12: 4th Chemotherapy Treatment.....................194
A Word About Sex During Chemotherapy 204
October 3: 5th Chemo Treatment 205
October 21: Another Surgical Consult 209
October 24: 6th (and Final) Chemo Treatment..................211

November 12: 2nd Stage Reconstruction 217
November 18: Dr. Da Lio Post Operative Appointment 220
November 21: Radiation Consult/Simulation 225
November 25: Dr. Chap Follow-up 229
December 3: Radiation Begins 231
December 17: The Occupational Therapist 233
Radiation Continues 235
January 15: The Final Treatment 238

Epilogue I 241

Epilogue II – Cancer for Two Two 244

Appendix 1: "Chris-isms" 247
Appendix 2: "Dave-isms" 249
Appendix 3: Fascinating (?) Facts 250
Appendix 4: Reasons Why Cancer Was a "Gift" 251
Appendix 5: Good Things About Having No Hair 253
Appendix 6: Tips for the Part-Time Caregiver 254
Appendix 7: Tips for Recording Doctor Visits 261
Appendix 8: Tips for Reducing Stress 263

Index 265

About the Author

Since 1982 Dave Balch worked from home where he developed, sold, and supported proprietary computer software for the corporate market. It was a successful business but he got burned out on software so he recently embarked on a speaking career. As part of that effort, he adopted the moniker of "The Stay-at-Home CEO™" and started a free newsletter called "Big Bucks in a Bathrobe" delivered by email, which has thousands of subscribers in over 30 countries (as of this writing). He also developed a web site (www.TheStayAtHomeCEO.com) with the mission of helping small business owners who want to "Make More Money and Have More Fun" with their small businesses.

(As a result of his caregiving experience, however, Dave no longer pursues The Stay-at-Home CEO in order to concentrate on helping other cancer patients and their families. This new career is described on page 243.)

He and his wife, Christine Trammell Balch, a homemaker, have essentially been together 24 hours a day, 7 days a week for all of this time and have probably spent more time together than couples who have been married 60 years!

They live in absolute paradise: in the San Bernardino Mountains of Southern California about 90 miles east of Los Angeles. In 1997 they built a small ranch where they now live with their animal "children:" two horses, two dogs, two cats, three fish, and a really mean parrot. (We must clarify here: Chris has had this parrot since 1957 and they grew up together. He had his adult feathers when they got him, so he was at least five years old at the time, and they believe that he was snatched from the jungle and taken away from his mate. Chris adores this bird and the bird seems to adore her as well, but he is mean to everybody else. Considering his probable past, who could blame him??)

Dave and Chris have always been very healthy. With the horses, walking the dogs up and down slopes in the forest, and taking care of the property (which is at an elevation of 5,800 feet), their lifestyle in the mountains requires much more exercise on a daily basis than most people normally get. (Visiting friends have told them that the walk from the barn to the house, which is uphill, was difficult for them; Dave and Chris have to do it at least four times a day!) Plus, Chris has always been careful with her diet, subscribing to several health magazines and newsletters. She is aware of what is good for her and what isn't and, with rare exceptions, eats a very healthy diet. Her active life has given her a terrific figure and she is in excellent physical condition, which made the breast cancer diagnosis all the more surprising.

Other than his wife and animals, Dave's main interests are motorcycling and total eclipses of the sun, which you will learn more about later.

Acknowledgements

Friends/Relatives

Barbara Balch (my sister): thank you so much for your incredible contribution to this project, even though it put a great deal of stress on you and your schedule. Your amazing cover design touches everyone who sees it.

Georgia Leynaert (Chris's sister): thank you for your many hours of editing and feedback, and for your wonderful support at so many of Chris's appointments and procedures. You were a great source of joy and comfort to both of us.

John Trammell (Chris's brother) and Patty Kreymborg: your visits lifted everyone's spirits.

Kate Helfman (my assistant and our dear friend): how can we ever thank you for all you did and the sacrifices you made in order to support us during this difficult time? If it hadn't been for you, Chris would not have been able to be sick!

Anne Bellegia and Terry Asnes (dear friends): if it weren't for your nagging, uh, I mean encouragement and advice, we may have never gotten that second opinion and found UCLA and their fantastic doctors. Just imagine how different the outcome of all this might have been. Thank you for that, and for the wonderful massages you arranged for us, the incredible flowers you sent, and for the wonderful meals you thoughtfully brought us from The Claim Jumper.

Kathy Walsh (E.R. Nurse, next-door neighbor, and wonderful all-around person): maker of the most incredible enchiladas, and my medical backup. It was comforting to know you were there, and willing to drop everything at anytime if we needed you, which we did on more than one occasion!

Kendall S. Wagner, M.D. (friend since the 9ᵗʰ grade): thank you for your caring and for your thoughtful and intelligent medical advice and guidance.

Dr. Gail Steger and Dr. Sonia Riha ("honorary aunts"): always there with a kind word, many gifts to lift our spirits, and great companionship. Gail, we miss you every day. Sonia, we hope we can be as much comfort to you as you were to us and to Gail in her final days.

Kim Willman (Chris's manicurist [and "Life Advisor"]): always cheerful, so many wonderful caring cards and notes, and helping Chris to feel her beautiful and feminine best.

Dale Purcell (hair stylist) and Glen Thompson (friend): for the most outrageous and wonderful diversion that brought so much joy and laughter to so many people, namely the Carmen Miranda hat. Thank you, thank you, thank you!

Shelly Dayan (friend): thank you so much for helping to keep our horses healthy, and for the hundreds of pounds of manure that you picked up for us!

Karen Hanson, Mandy Mc Andrew (friends): thank you for your wonderful food and for helping with the horses, including manure patrol.

Tamara Jones, Karen Baldwin (friends): thank you for bringing food, make that "great" food!

John and Linda Farley (friends): thank you for all the laughs in radiation, and for the great apple pie!

Becci Ripson (new friend): thank you for your positive attitude and imagery.

Office of Kyi Kyi (Gigi) Win, M.D.

You were all so wonderful and accommodating throughout the entire experience, especially when Chris was in the middle of chemo and needed to avoid the public.

Gigi Win, M.D.
Gilda Galvan, receptionist
Gina Morek, R.N.
Lee Karpinski, R.N.

UCLA Medical Center,
UCLA Department of Medicine,
UCLA Revlon/UCLA Breast Center,
UCLA Division of Plastic and Reconstructive Surgery,
UCLA Santa Monica Hematology/Oncology Group,
UCLA Division of Surgical Oncology

We simply cannot say enough good things about UCLA! Without exception, everyone we encountered was pleasant, skilled at their profession, and knew our case and what had to be done. The coordination between departments, doctors, and other personnel was impressive; when it came to Chris's care, everyone seemed to know what everyone else was doing. It was an incredible experience of medicine at its finest. We can't thank you enough. Unfortunately there are many, many people whose names we simply do not know, but you know who you are and this "thank you" goes to you as well!

Mai N. Brooks, M.D., Surgical Oncologist
Andrew L. Da Lio, M.D., F.A.C.S, Plastic Surgeon
Linnea A. Chap, M.D., Hematology Oncologist
Rosa Mendez, L.V.N.
Iris Isla, Chemotherapy Nurse
Joan Messina, Chemotherapy Nurse
Pete Zimak, Pharmacy Technician
Fern Robinson, Medical Assistant
Jo Jenkins, Administrative Assistant
Debra Parson, Administrative Assistant
Tammie Tillmon, Administrative Assistant
Tina Hoff, Chemotherapy Nurse
Susan Sanceri, Chemotherapy Nurse
Miguel Cardenas, Administrative Assistant
Leah Bailey, Chemotherapy Nurse

Loma Linda University Hospital, Dept. of Radiation Medicine
Loma Linda University Medical Center, Outpatient Rehabilitation Center

You were all kind, caring, and comforting during a difficult time. It was always a pleasure to see your smiling faces day after day after day after day after day after day...

Janet M. Hocko, M.D., Assistant Professor of Radiation Medicine
Irene Bielitz, R.N.
Renato Farias, Radiation Therapist
Devon Elston-Hurdle, Radiation Therapist
Vickie Utt, Radiation Therapist
Dale James, Radiation Therapist
Deanna Stires, Radiation Therapist
Kimberly A. Wood, Senior Occupational Therapist CDT

Mastermind Group

Thank you all for your caring, understanding, and messages of support.

Farla Binder	*Maura Raffensperger*
Geoff Bryan	*Steve Stewart*
Roger Burgraff	*Constance Yambert*

National Speakers Association

I've never known such a wonderful organization of friendly, caring, and helpful people.

Greg Godek	*Nancy Miller*
Judith Parker Harris	*Mike Rounds*
Judy Jernudd	*Alexandra Sagerman*
Darlene March	*Karyn Buxman*

Sandy Chetelat, Blue Jay Physical Therapy

Thank you for having the insight to suggest the MRI of Chris's hip when you did. There's no telling how this might have turned out had we waited.

Kari Enge, M.D. Psychiatry: thank you for your caring and training in Guided Imagery.

Introduction

"You have cancer."

There had been some small talk and then Dr. Win finally just blurted it out. I heard myself say a very bad word that begins with "F" but no one seemed to notice. I was a little embarrassed, though, about using such language in front of these two ladies. I knew we were about to embark on one hellava ride, but really had no idea of the extent of that ride.

Chris had discovered the lump 12 days earlier while taking a shower. Not one to shy away from bad news, she went in the very next day for an exam and Dr. Win said she didn't think it was anything to worry about but that she should have a biopsy to be sure. (A "biopsy" is a procedure where they extract a small portion of the lump and examine it under a microscope.) Due to a frustrating set of circumstances beyond anyone's control, we had to wait a week until the biopsy could be performed at a hospital about 45 minutes' drive from our home. The results of that biopsy had just come in, and the doctor had called us to come in to her office at 8:00 that evening; that was our first clue that the news was not good. (It was April 22, our 19th wedding anniversary).

After the bad news had been delivered, the doctor, a small lady from Burma, said, "Let's pray," and the three of us joined hands. She asked for guidance for all of the doctors and nurses that would be taking care of Chris and I was choking back tears, not only for the fear of the unknowns ahead and for the sorrow for Chris, but because I was so touched at the kind gesture from this gentle lady.

After the prayer Chris said, "Look at the clock!" It was 8:20, which was exactly the time of day that we were married, and on the 19th anniversary of that day as well! It was very strange to think that when we got married, it would be *ex-*

"Nothing has been exaggerated, embellished, or fabricated; as you will see, there was no need."

---

actly 19 years later, *to the minute,* that we would get this life-changing news.

As we walked outside, Chris was deep in thought (or was it shock?). I didn't know what to say to her, but I desperately wanted to comfort her in some way. We let the dogs out of the car so they could run around and I told her, "I'm so, so sorry. I want you to know that you are NOT alone, and that I will be with you every step of the way."

And so began the big adventure. This book is the true story of exactly what happened, why we did what we did and, most importantly, what I learned about caregiving for the most important person in my life. Nothing has been exaggerated, embellished, or fabricated; as you will see, there was no need.

It is a story of teamwork, exceptional courage, top doctors, medical miracles, priorities, humor, and lots and lots of driving. It is my hope that in it you find courage and inspiration that will help you with your own cancer battle, or, for that matter, any other battle you may face.

The single most important thing that we did when we first got the diagnosis was to learn as much as we could, as quickly as we could. Herein lies a basic truth, and it applies to both the patient and the caregiver. In fact, it is a basic truth of life. The more you know about something scary, the less scary it becomes. Put another, perhaps more familiar way: information is power. The more information you have about something, the more power you feel you have over it.

This was true for Chris's brother and sister, and it was also true for us. When Chris was first diagnosed, we knew nothing about cancer. It scared the hell out of us. But the more we found out about types of cancer and treatments, the less frightening it became. Even when the prospects are unpleasant, they are not as intimidating when you know what they are and you can stare them in the face.

Why the title "Cancer for Two?" Because breast cancer, or any cancer for that matter, *dramatically* affects the partner as well as the patient. If you, as partner, think that it's a shame that she has cancer but that your life will continue on just as it has in the past with a few minor inconveniences, you are in for a rude awakening. Whether you like it or not, whether you want it or not, your world is going to be in chaos for a while. It is important to remember that the chaos is not a permanent condition, but you will deal with chaos for a while regardless.

Remember that we're talking life-threatening disease here and, at the same time, entering a world of medical terms and procedures that is very foreign to most of us. Either of these situations is frightening enough; combine them and the stress of coping is considerable.

There are a million things to do and deal with, many of which can be pretty scary. This is the time to step up to the plate and do as many of the things that you *can* do, to free up her energy to battle the disease, which is obviously something you *cannot* do. Coordinate scheduling and appointments as much as possible so she doesn't have to. Provide or arrange for transportation so she doesn't have to. Keep the house clean, take care of the children and pets, make the

"The single most important thing we did when we first got the diagnosis was to learn as much as we could, as quickly as we could."

> "It was her job to get better. It was my job
> to do everything else."

meals, buy the groceries, etc. so she doesn't have to. It is, perhaps more than at any other time in your lives, a battle for *both* of you; it is truly "Cancer for Two."

I am proud to say that I went with Chris to every single appointment and procedure from the biopsy in April through the radiation consult and simulation in November. I made all of the appointments, maintained the schedule, did most of the driving, took care of the ranch and animals when she couldn't, cooked when I had to, bought the groceries, kept our friends and family informed, dealt with insurance and finances, and generally did everything possible to eliminate for her whatever stress and worry I could and provide her with love and encouragement. It was her job to get better. It was my job to do everything else.

This is what worked for us; your patient may *prefer* to do some of these things. If so, let her! This isn't about power; it's about reducing stress and providing love and support. If your patient feels more in control if she does a lot of the work herself, then you are *creating* stress by doing these things for her, not reducing it. In Chris's case, she felt powerless and it helped her feel like she had *some* control over *something* to at least drive some of the time. And so she did.

You will have to put parts of your life on hold for a while, make sacrifices, and do some things you don't want to do. Do them anyway. It's the right thing to do. Mark Twain once said, *"Do the right thing; it will surprise some people and astonish the rest!"*

Think of it as an investment in your relationship and your life. (Besides, if you ever get a serious illness she'll owe you big time!)

It is my intention to share many of the lessons that I learned from this experience and it is my hope that these lessons will help you get through your own challenges. I know that it would have helped me to have this information as soon as possible. The lessons I learned were not only about cancer itself, but about thoughtful caregiving, about myself, and about other people as well.

I will tell you right now that, although I certainly would rather that Chris hadn't gotten sick, the fact that she did gave me the opportunity of a lifetime. It was the opportunity to experience the unbridled joy of taking care of the most important person in my life and to help her through this ordeal, a joy that brings tears to my eyes even as I write this. To see her sleeping with her cute little bald head, knowing that she is safe and warm and in my care, gave me a feeling that all is well with the world in spite of her illness, and that I am doing something that is truly meaningful and important.

Put aside your fear and embrace this opportunity to make a huge difference in the life of someone that is important to you.

Put aside petty differences, because your job now is to help her through it, not to "be right." Let things go; nothing is more important than reducing the stress on your patient, and if that means overlooking something rather than starting an argument, so be it. Whatever it is, it probably isn't important enough to justify the burden of the conflict. And, if it *is* that important, *let it go anyway.*

The main thing, the *only* thing, is to create the most positive environment possible. Never underestimate the healing power of a good attitude on the part of your patient; the easier you make her life and the less she has to worry about, the better her attitude will be and, in my opinion, the better the outcome will be.

Do you see how important your role is?

Laugh. Cry. Care. It's a feeling like no other.

Be smart. Be thoughtful. Be careful.

Internet Extras and Services

www.CancerForTwo.com is an integral part of this book, including:

- video clips and color photos *
- an easy way to order additional copies of *Cancer for Two* with a free bonus available only for Internet orders: you can immediately download the electronic version of *Cancer for Two*.

Be sure to also visit *The Patient/Partner Project* website at **www.ThePatientPartnerProject.org** to take advantage of free information and services for patients and partners:

- Free online progress reporting keeps your family and friends updated without stressful and time-consuming phone calls, telling the same stories and answering the same questions over and over. Post your progress reports right on the website; then our system will send an email to all registered family and friends to tell them that there is news. Simple and secure; no one can read your postings unless they know your private and unique MemberID, chosen by you.
- Free e-mail mini-courses. (A "mini-course" is a series of emails sent automatically, each containing an article on a specific topic, such as coping strategies.)

The Patient/Partner Project is proud to be a member of the National Quality Caregiving Coalition (NQCC) of the Rosalynn Carter Institute.

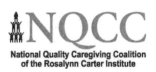

*To complete your *Cancer for Two* reading and sharing experience, visit **www.CancerForTwo.com/c42book** where you can see the photos and video clips of people and places mentioned within these pages. This private area of the website cannot be accessed from anywhere else on the site: it is available only to those who have this exact address.

April 10:
The Lump and Biopsy

It was evening and I was in the kitchen when Chris came in and said, "I found a lump." She had been in the shower and, as she often does, was doing a self-exam when she found it.

The lump was on the top center of her right breast, and it felt pretty large and firm. I was reminded of the lump she had found about two years earlier, which had also appeared suddenly. In that case, she had had it examined immediately and they determined that it was just a cyst, but they removed fluid from the lump and sent it to the lab just to be sure. I couldn't help but remember how the surgeon had allowed me to be in the room when he inserted what seemed like a very large needle directly into the lump and withdrew the fluid. Yikes! He stuck a needle into her breast! That has to be a pretty sensitive area, and Chris didn't even flinch, showing her mettle and how tough she was. (As it turns out, that was just a preview of things to come.) I could only identify with a needle inserted into a similarly sensitive area of my own body. It was a very colorful scene: the fluid was green and I was blue.

Based on that memory, however, and the fact that I am a die-hard optimist, I told her, "It's probably just another cyst. I'm sure it will be fine." (In retrospect, I think that part of my optimism was based on the "bad-things-happen-to-other-people-but-not-us" mentality, which made the concept of it actually being cancer beyond the realm of my imagination.)

The next day she called for a walk-in appointment with Dr. Win, our local family physician; a cute, tiny, bubbly lady from Burma who is always kind and caring. The appointment was made for late afternoon. Unfortunately, I had a meeting

> "... part of my optimism was based on the 'bad-things-happen-to-other-people-but-not-us' mentality. . ."

in the city and would be gone all day so I couldn't go with Chris, but I intended to keep in touch by cell phone.

When I was finished with my meeting, I was hoping for a message on the cell phone saying that all was well; there was none. I tried to call Chris but was unsuccessful, so I went ahead with my plans to see Ken (a dear friend from middle school) and his new home, then go to dinner with him and his girlfriend. As we sat in the restaurant, I tried to reach Chris several times. Each time I couldn't, I got more worried.

I finally reached her as dinner was being served, and I found myself talking on a cell phone in a restaurant while my table companions just sat there. I felt like I was being incredibly rude; I am always annoyed when I see people talking on a cell phone in a restaurant. (Maybe next time I'll have a little more compassion for them; after all, they, too, may be having an emergency!)

Chris told me that Dr. Win didn't like the way the lump felt and wanted her to have a biopsy, even though she was pretty sure it was benign, and that her office would call the next day to arrange for an appointment in the city. I was not happy to hear this news; I wanted to hear that Dr. Win had said, "Ah, it's nothing; go home, have some chicken soup, it'll be gone in the morning!" Or something like that.

When I got off the phone my friends could see that I was a little distressed, and Ken gave me a pep talk. As a leading orthopedic surgeon in the area he knew lots of quality medical professionals that could help us if necessary.

"I can hook you up with the best people in the area," he assured me. "She will get the best care possible."

The next day was a flurry of frustrations as the biopsy appointment was made for April 19th, one week later, at a hospital in the city. A *week*?? I wanted to have it done that day! As it turned out, this was going to be an ultrasound-guided biopsy, which means that an ultrasound device is used to get an image of the lump on a screen, which they then use to guide the needle that extracts the tissue from the lump. They had two such ultrasound machines, but one of them was not operational and wouldn't be until the following week, which played havoc with their schedule. I tried calling supervisors but they could do nothing either, so Friday the 19th it would be.

We arrived for the biopsy on time, which is no small accomplishment for us. We were both a little nervous and we both wanted me to be in the room when he did the procedure. Unfortunately, the doctor wouldn't allow it because he said that he had had too much trouble in the past with spouses who wanted to watch and then couldn't handle it; he ended up spending too much time tending to *their* needs. So I sat in the waiting room trying to work on my laptop computer and Chris appeared about 30 minutes later, seemingly none the worse for wear. They told us we would have results by Monday or Tuesday.

On the way home, she told me that they had used a gun-like device, which quickly inserted a needle and pulled it out again, presumably containing tissue from the lump. Several samples had been taken, and it was getting painful for her, but the doctor had stopped before it became unbearable. (At the time I thought she had been pretty brave, but "brave" would soon take on a whole new meaning.)

It seemed like the weekend dragged on and on, and we couldn't imagine that the results would be anything but, "It's benign, nothing to worry about."

April 22:
The Diagnosis

Monday was our 19th wedding anniversary (and also 24 years since we met), but the mood was somewhat subdued because we couldn't stop wondering about the biopsy. That afternoon we got a call from Dr. Win's office. She wanted Chris to come in at 8:00 that night, which pretty much told Chris all she needed to know.

We showed up a little before 8:00 and Chris was sure that the nurses, whom we all know (it's that small-town thing that we have up here in the mountains), were acting a little different than they normally do. It seemed that they had trouble making eye contact.

We were shown into the exam room and Dr. Win appeared, making some small talk and appearing, to me at least, to be a little uneasy. Chris was on my left and we were holding hands; Dr. Win was standing in front of us and to my right. Finally, there was a lull in the small talk; I saw a fleeting glimpse of sadness and resignation on the doctor's face as she took a deep breath and then softly blurted it out:

"You have cancer."

I was shocked to hear myself say, "Oh, fuck."

Chris said, "I knew it."

I couldn't see Chris's face because I was facing Dr. Win, and I was afraid to look.

"The biopsy shows that you have ductal carcinoma in situ, a fairly common form of breast cancer," Dr. Win explained, in our first of many experiences with the world of medical mumbo jumbo.

"What the heck does that really mean?" I asked her.

She proceeded to tell us about milk ducts and cancer and the term "in situ" (pronounced "in SIGH to") which means that it is contained within the ducts, which was a good thing.

To my surprise, she pulled up a chair directly in front of us and said, "Let's pray." We all joined hands and she said a short prayer for Chris and for all of the medical personnel that would be taking care of her. I was very touched by this sweet gesture and was choking back tears.

When we finished, Chris looked at the clock and said, "Look at the time!" It was 8:20, the exact time that we had been married 19 years earlier. We had chosen that time for the ceremony because 5 years before that, on that same date and at that same time, we had met. (We were also standing on the exact spot in a local disco *where* we had met. Ain't it romantic?) How strange that we should get this life-changing news *exactly* 19 years (to the minute) after we were married.

Since it has always been my basic instinct to take care of and protect Chris, I felt the need to take charge of the situation as I had in previous family emergencies. I asked Dr. Win, "What's next?"

She said that we needed to find a surgeon that specializes in these things to remove the lump and find out more about the nature of the cancer. I figured that my friend Ken would be one of my first calls when we got home.

Not too much was said until we got into the parking lot. We had brought Simone and Emma, our two black standard poodles, (any excuse for a ride in the car) and we let them out so they could run around a little. We followed them with plastic bags in hand, both of us lost in thought, perhaps even in shock. I couldn't help but think, "Oh my God, she could actually *die.*" It was unthinkable. This is the sort of thing that happens to other people, or in the movies, *but not to us.*

Even though we were walking in silence, I noticed that all of my senses were heightened. We were holding hands and her hand seemed warmer and softer, the air seemed crisper, the sky darker, and the noises of the night seemed sharper. It

> ## ". . . I want you to know that you won't be alone. I will be with you every step of the way."

was my first taste of a phenomenon that I would notice many more times in the coming weeks

I couldn't begin to imagine what was racing through Chris's mind, but I wanted to comfort her in any way I could.

"I'm so, so sorry that you have to go through this, Chris, but I want you to know that you won't be alone. I will be with you every step of the way."

She thanked me and said that she knew that, but was relatively quiet as we watched the dogs romping in the grass without a care in the world.

When we got home, we headed for separate phones. Because I work at home, I've installed a small business phone system in the house with 5 outside lines and 10 individual phones, including 2 in the barn. It's a great system, perfect for us. That's how we could both go for the phone at the same time; we talked on separate lines.

Chris called Georgia, her sister, and I called Jane Hill, who is a friend of mine from the Los Angeles Chapter of the National Speakers Association. (After 20 years in a home software business, I had decided to change careers and had become "The Stay-at-Home CEO™," helping small and home businesses through speaking and on the Internet. I had joined the National Speakers Association and its local chapter to learn as much as I could about the speaking business.) Belonging to that organization brings me in contact with many interesting and diverse people who speak on an incredible range of topics. Jane's topic is a humorous look at breast cancer and she, herself, was a breast cancer survivor, so calling her was a natural... "What should I do?"

> **"Bring a tape recorder to all doctor appointments. If the doctor won't allow you to record. . . get another doctor."**

Fortunately Jane answered the phone, and referred me to several web sites and told me that I could call on her anytime for advice and support. She was very comforting and helpful and gave me a truly outstanding piece of advice: bring a tape recorder to all doctor appointments. If the doctor won't allow you to record the conversation, get another doctor. (See the Appendix titled "Tips for Recording Doctor Appointments" for some detailed suggestions on how best to do just that; there's more to it than you might think.) She also sent me about 5 pounds of books and other materials.

My next call was to Ken, who was mortified at the news. He told me about a couple of surgeons at his hospital that specialize in breast cancer, and gave me their names and phone numbers. I asked him, "If it were your wife, which one would you call?"

He thought about it for a moment and said, "Dr. Loman." *(Author's note: "Dr. Loman" is not his real name.)*

After that I called Barbara, my sister, who lives in New York City, as well as several other friends.

After spending considerable time at the web sites that Jane recommended, I was running on information overload. So much to learn, so many new terms, and so many variables, plus I didn't know which ones applied to Chris's situation because, at this point, we didn't know very much about breast cancer in general or her tumor in particular. My anxiety level was rising to barely tolerable levels and I was up very late that night.

As difficult as those moments were, looking back on it now I realize that it was absolutely the best thing I could have done. As I mentioned in the introduction, it is imperative that you learn as much as you can as quickly as you can in order to reduce your fear of the unknown. It is a classic example of the adage "information is power" because the more we learned the less apprehensive we were, *even if what we learned was scary.*

In the meantime, Chris spent a considerable amount of time on another line talking first to her sister, Georgia, then to her brother, John. (Georgia lives about 100 miles from us in an ocean community near Los Angeles, and John lives 450 miles away in a city that is 30 miles east of San Francisco.) They were both astonished that Chris, of all people, could have cancer because a) there is no history of breast cancer in their family and b), Chris was so active, so health conscious, and, well, just so darned healthy! How could this be? Chris eats salmon and broccoli for breakfast for heavens' sake!!

John, in a mock fit of guilt, told Chris how sorry he was that he broke her finger on the wagon, referring to a child-hood incident where he dragged her around in his red wagon.

"That's when the cancer started!" Chris told him, jokingly implying that the cancer was, in fact, his fault. They both had a good laugh. The news was barely an hour old and the humor was already starting. There is no better way to diffuse the worry and anxiety than to laugh about some aspect of the problem.

We have no human children, but we do have a large number of animals (read that as "menagerie") that are like children to us. At this writing, we have two horses, two dogs, two cats, two fish, and a really mean parrot. We cater to their every need and put their needs before ours a large majority of the time. I do love them intensely, but Chris is much more of a fanatic (read that as "mildly neurotic") about them than I am.

" . . . it is imperative that you learn as much as you can as quickly as you can. "

A very important facet of our relationship, which proved to be a crucial element in this story, is that we laugh a lot. We laugh at each other, at ourselves, and at everything else as well. Silliness is a big part of our interaction, and most of that silliness is related to our animals. Each animal has a "voice", which we then use to tell each other what we think that that animal would be saying if it could. For example, Simone is a standard French poodle, so her "voice" has an outrageous French accent.

"Mamá, I zink zat you should take me in ze car, toot suite!"

This whole talking-for-the-animals silliness actually serves a vital purpose in our relationship. Whenever one of us makes a mistake or does something that would be easy for the other to criticize, *the criticism comes from an animal (using that animal's voice) instead of from one of us.* As strange as it may seem, if it comes in an animal's voice it somehow isn't offensive and it's a good way for us to tease each other and laugh about it at the same time.

For example, after a day in the city I forgot to get gas and when Chris needed that car the next day it was practically running on fumes. When she got back, she came into my office and said (in Simone's voice), "Papá, you left ze car wis no gas for mamá. Why did you do zis zing? I know bettair zen zat and I am only a dog!" I apologized (by telling Simone to tell "Mamá" I was sorry) and we both laughed about it.

Imagine how different it would have been if Chris had come in and said, "Thanks a lot. You left the car with no gas, so I was late because I had to stop and get some!"

Lily, one of our cats, had a problem because, at one time, we had too many cats in the house. Cats are very territorial

---

"There is no better way to diffuse the worry and anxiety than to laugh about some aspect of the problem."

---

and each has a limit as to how many other cats they will tolerate. Lily is a two-cat cat, which we unfortunately discovered after we got a third cat. Lily reacted by urinating in the house, which is a *very* bad thing. Few substances on earth are as toxic and as permanent as cat urine.

The reason that I mention this problem is that we began to call Lily "The Urinator" and her "voice" is modeled after that of Arnold Schwarzenneger who is known for his movie role as "The Terminator." We also threw in a little Elmer Fudd just for fun. (Believe it or not, this will be relevant in just a minute.)

"I *am* da yawinata, so don't make me mad or I will yawinate on you or on sumfing you twezure!"

As we were getting ready for bed the night we got the diagnosis, Lily walked in the room. She said (courtesy of yours truly), "New mommy, I huwd about what da docta said. It *IS* a tuma!" (This was a reference to Kindergarten Cop, a movie in which Arnold Schwarzenegger ends up teaching a class of kindergarteners. He told the kids he had a headache and one of them suggested that it might be a tumor. "It's not a tuma!" he told them in his wonderful Austrian accent; a very funny scene that we refer to whenever we can.)

Lily continued her thoughts about the tumor, "...and I'm gonna yawinate on it until it goes away!"

It was my first attempt at humor in the face of this news and I knew I was taking a chance, but it did break the tension. We had a good laugh and we both felt a little better. (*I* did, anyway... I'm pretty sure she did too.)

At 8:30 the next morning I was on the phone with Dr. Loman's office and was thrilled to find out that he had an opening for 9:00 a.m. the very next day. Perfect: we didn't have to wait! He would need a few things, however. He wanted to see Chris's most recent mammograms, and he wanted to see the biopsy report. Great; more things to do. I made a few phone calls and had the biopsy report faxed to me that afternoon. I called the local hospital to see what we needed to do in order to get the mammograms, so they faxed me an authorization form for Chris to sign.

At this point it's important to note that we live in the San Bernardino Mountains of Southern California about 90 miles east of Los Angeles. Our elevation of 5,800 feet (approximately 1800 meters) is absolute paradise to us: we have clean air, heavily forested solitude, and no congestion. Local medical facilities, however, are limited; come to think of it, most everything is limited up here and that's the way we like it. That fact, however, plays an extremely important part in our overall experience because of the distances involved. Going "down the hill" (read "to the city") meant a minimum of 30 minutes of curvy mountain roads just to get to the beginning of civilization; most medical facilities are much farther than that.

We had two cars: a 13-year-old Nissan 2-seater sports car, and a 10-year-old Toyota 4Runner, which is a 4-seater SUV with an enclosed cargo area behind the passenger seats. We used the Toyota (we call it "the truck" because it is really an SUV on a pickup truck frame) for most of the driving because Chris was often very tired from dealing with her illness and there was plenty of room for Chris to sleep comfortably in the back. We did take the 2-seater a couple of times when the truck was being repaired. (During this ordeal, we joked that our next car was going to be an ambulance!)

I bring this up because Dr. Loman's office was in Orange County, which is about 75 miles away (that translates into 90 minutes of driving). We decided to spend the night nearby so we wouldn't have to worry about traffic and could actually get to the appointment on time.

Staying overnight anywhere, however, can be quite a challenge for us because of all of our animals. This situation is no small part of this entire story, and here's why. First of all, we are very particular about how our animal family is cared for. (People who know us will laugh out loud at the previous sentence as the understatement of the century.)

With few exceptions, when visitors first see how our animals live they tell us that when they die they want to come back as one of our pets. They get my standard reply, "Okay, but there's a waiting list!"

Secondly, we have a variety of different types of animals that must be cared for by someone who knows about that type of animal. The fish are easiest; for a single night we can just leave 'em! The parrot is easy too; make sure he'll be warm and that he has plenty of seeds. Cats are no problem; leave some dry food and a clean litter box and we're good to go. The dogs are a little more difficult, but we have several friends with dogs who feel about them the way we feel about ours. (Although more things to do, it would be simple to drop them off for the night and pick them up the next day.)

The horses, however, are another story. Not only do they have to stay on the property, but whoever takes care of them has to know about horses. It's not as easy as simply throwing some hay on the ground and shoveling the manure, especially *our* horses, who require special supplements and other care. Besides, horses are, in spite of their size, deceptively fragile animals and a serious situation could arise that would look completely normal to someone who doesn't know about such things.

We have found that the best way, the only way, to solve this problem is to have someone whom we really trust stay in the house and take care of everyone.

Meet Kate, my assistant who has worked in our home office for 11 years as of this writing. Kate is, in a word, wonderful. She is always cheerful, fiercely loyal, happy to help in any way she can, and loves our animals almost as much as we do. One word from us and she'll drop almost anything to help. She and Alan, her husband, literally move into our home when we need them to (vacations, for example) and so it was with this situation. She said, "Don't worry about a thing, we'll take care of everyone." What a relief! It was the first of what

"... 'on the roller coaster of life, I guess it's my turn to be in the front car.'"

turned out to be many times that Kate would come to our rescue with animal-care duty.

Later that day, I took the signed authorization form to our local hospital to get Chris's mammograms. On the way home, I stopped at a market where they sell individual flowers so you can make your own bouquet. I picked out a number of Chris's favorites (but no yellow... she doesn't like yellow) and brought them home to surprise her. She loved the flowers, but even more she loved the fact that I picked the assortment myself with her in mind.

While arranging the flowers in a vase, Chris told me that she had been thinking about the whole situation. She told me, "I look at this way: on the roller coaster of life, I guess it's my turn to be in the front car. Bring it on! I've always wondered what I'd look like with no hair."

'Atta boy, girl! What a great attitude! My heart soared like an eagle. That statement is just one of many inspiring things that she said during the course of her treatment; see the Appendix titled "Chris-isms" for more of them.

We realized that we had some uncharted waters ahead, and that each of us would have things to do that we've never done before so we had a talk about how we were going to handle the situation. In the normal course of our life together we have a deal: I make all the phone calls (she doesn't like the phone), she writes all the cards and letters (I hate to write cards and letters). This would be no exception, which meant that I would be handling all of the scheduling of appointments and keeping everyone informed about her progress. Plus, I would be taking care of the animals and other household chores when she was unable to.

"You're going to have to help me help you," I told her, "by lightening up a bit on how everything has to be done around here." (Chris likes everything to be "just so" and there isn't much wiggle room, especially when it comes to the comfort and happiness of the animals and the house being clean.) "I'll do the best I can, but we have to keep our priorities in mind and, as long as everybody stays healthy, it's going to have to be okay if I cut some corners."

She understood exactly what I meant and promised to do her best, but she knows how she is when it comes to the animals and knew that would not be easy for her.

Then she said, "…and you're going to have to give me a break if I snap at you because I'm not feeling well." She was referring to my super-sensitivity to her tone of voice; she is a more emotional person than I am and sometimes expresses herself strongly (it's the Irish in her, I guess). If it is anger or frustration she is expressing, I am usually quick to take it personally because, after all, I am a man and my knee-jerk reaction to most of these outbursts is that it is my responsibility to fix whatever is wrong. If I can step back from the situation and see that what she is expressing has nothing to do with me it is easier to handle, but after 24 years with her I still forget to do that and then I get my feelings hurt or my anxiety level soars. We have learned that one way to help me handle this is for her to remind me by saying something like, "I'm not mad at you but…" Now Chris was telling me, in advance, that she will probably get cranky because of how she is feeling and that if she does it has nothing to do with me and I shouldn't take it personally, even if she doesn't 'warn' me in advance.

It was a meaningful, intimate conversation in that we each expressed our needs to the other and asked for help and cooperation in doing what had to be done in these difficult circumstances. This 90-second discussion made a tremendous difference in our relationship for the next nine months, in that we gave each other "permission" to have faults and asked each other for what we needed. I talk more about this sort of thing in the next chapter "*Giving Permission.*"

Fair enough: a lot had been said in a short time and I knew that it would be a rough road. Not only were there all of the animals to take care of, there was the house, the property, grocery shopping, cooking, and, oh yes, *making some money*! Part of my Stay-at-Home CEO business was a bi-weekly newsletter sent by e-mail, along with a weekly column in a local newspaper and a bi-weekly spot on our local cable channel. I was also working on a book and some other products, and I wasn't sure how I was going to be able to keep up with what I started, not to mention finding the time to accept speaking engagements and develop the products. Fortunately, we had some residual income from the software business that met about 75% of our needs, but now we would be taking on our portion of the medical expenses in addition to everything else.

Speaking of medical expenses, I started to wonder what all of this was going to cost and how much our insurance would cover. I called our insurance carrier, Blue Cross of California, and asked them. Our plan is a "PPO" (Preferred Provider Organization) which means that they contract with various doctors and hospitals that are willing to agree to Blue Cross's payment schedule and other restrictions, a situation that benefits everyone involved. The benefit to the doctors is that they will attract Blue Cross patients. The benefit to Blue Cross is that they get discounted rates on services. The benefit to the patients is that they get a wide variety of doctors and hospitals to choose from; "anybody who's anybody" accepts Blue Cross, so we could go almost wherever we wanted for treatment and it would be covered.

Blue Cross told me that as long as we go to doctors that

" . . . we each expressed our needs to the other and asked for help and cooperation in doing what had to be done in these difficult circumstances."

---

are under their contract I don't have to worry. Our deductible was $1,500; after that they pay 75% and we pay 25% until we have paid a total of $4,000, including the deductible, in a given calendar year. After that, they pay 100% for the remainder of the year. (That is the way *our* policy is written; every policy is different, however, so be sure to check carefully with your own carrier.)

I am happy to say that that was the only time I needed to talk to Blue Cross during the entire course of Chris's treatment. When Blue Cross approvals were needed, the doctors' offices requested and got them. The medical facilities submitted the bills and Blue Cross paid their share. Period. If there were disputes, I didn't hear about them. I didn't hear so much as a peep; after all the bad press that health insurance has gotten, I was very pleasantly surprised. There is enough to worry about when you have to deal with a major illness; the last thing I needed was to fight with my medical insurance. Although I didn't realize it at the time, our insurance was to become a non-issue, just like it should have been.

Based on this new information, I started calculating what my portion of the medical expenses was going to be. It was still early in the year (end of April), I wondered if Chris's entire treatment would be completed in the same calendar year in which it began so I wouldn't be subject to another deductible the next year. I realized that we could have a situation where there were several options that were the same medically but different financially depending on the timing of the treatment. If such a situation came up, it was important to know how the coverage worked in order to make a good decision. At the time I pondered these questions, however, we didn't know enough about her course of treatment to determine the answers.

Insurance and financing were important to be aware of in order to be prepared, but I would never have considered compromising Chris's treatment in any way for any reason, including financial reasons.

> **"... if you take the trouble to look, you *can* find hope in the situation."**

We were as philosophic and positive about the situation as we could be. We tried to find some good things, given the situation, to focus on and this is what we came up with:

1. Chris gets regular checkups and had had a clean mammogram seven months earlier.

2. Chris caught it early – she does self-exams often and, when she found the lump, took immediate action rather than ignore it hoping it would go away.

3. Chris was in excellent health and physical condition, which was encouraging to know because it indicated that she would respond well to treatment and that she would probably bounce back quickly.

4. It was early in the year, which meant that we would probably get most of the treatment finished in one calendar year. That translated to less cost to us because we would only have one year's deductible to meet. (As it turned out, two weeks' treatment spilled into the next year, which ended up costing us another entire deductible, but at this time we didn't know that would happen so I clung to the happy thought that it wouldn't.)

It just goes to show that if you take the trouble to look, you *can* find hope in the situation.

We also did everything we could to joke about the situation with others. Whenever Chris encountered someone who politely asked, "How are you?" she would tell them. "I have breast cancer. How are *you?*" The smile on her face and twinkle in her eye let them know that she was doing okay with it and somewhat lessened the shock of the news. When someone asked me how we were doing I would say, "We're doing our best to laugh and eat our way through it." The "eat our way through it" phrase was a reference to the comfort food we were eating in great quantities. I told them that I figured I had a choice between alcohol and eating as a way to cope with the situation, but that since I don't drink (never have) I was eating comfort food. And lots of it; at that point the comfort value of food had more importance to me that the nutritional value. I am normally a reasonably healthy eater, but I decided that I didn't need to stress about my diet on top of everything else, and "all bets were off." I don't necessarily recommend this strategy to everyone because bad eating habits take a toll in their own way, but that's what I did and I survived. (So far, anyway.)

In the beginning few weeks of Chris's treatment, I found myself so stressed that I had to make some changes in my environment. One of the first things I noticed was that most of the things on TV were too upsetting to watch. The news, which is full of murder and mayhem, was the first to go; I simply got too anxious while I was watching it. Even simple dramas or movies with the mildest plots raised my anxiety level, and I had to turn off just about everything except comedies. Even those were too much for me, though, if there was anything in the plotline that even hinted of some tension.

Poncho, Chris's parrot, had some noisy toys that I couldn't tolerate. Actually, I guess it would be more accurate to say that they were toys that Chris put near Poncho's cage for his amusement. For example, there was a 6-inch-high rubber demon (a Halloween toy) that shook violently and made horrific screaming noises for about 15 seconds whenever something set off its motion sensor. We had to turn it off and put it away because every time it went off I became extremely tense and upset. At any other time it would have been merely annoying, but with my current state of mind it made me crazy and a couple of times I almost, literally, stomped it to smithereens.

Giving Permission

I'm going to take a short break in our story to discuss something that is absolutely critical to the outcome of your own situation.

Looking back on our experience, and after hearing about the experiences of others, I am convinced that this is a time when both of you, the patient and the partner, have to give yourselves and each other *permission*.

Permission to share. First of all, you need to give yourselves permission to share your illness with family and friends. This is equally true of the patient as well as the partner. Although this didn't happen to us, I've heard about women who feel they must remain stoic and that being "brave" meant that they didn't ask anyone for help or sympathy, and didn't complain or "bore" everyone with the details of their treatment. There are four reasons that I believe that this is a mistake:

1. By doing everything yourself, including your normal activities, you are burdening yourself with a tremendous amount of unnecessary stress. There is no question that this additional stress will compromise your treatment and recovery. You simply will not and cannot respond to your treatments as well as you would in a lower-stress environment. In other words, by refusing to allow anyone to help you, you are giving the cancer an advantage that you don't want it to have.

"... give yourselves permission to share your illness."

This is a terribly difficult time in your life: there is no shame in asking for help. No one will think you are weak or incapable. I learned a very valuable lesson when I was young: it takes more courage to walk away from a fight than it does to actually fight. I remember being shocked at this basic concept, but immediately realized the truth in it. The same thing applies to asking for help: you may think that doing everything yourself takes courage, but it really takes more courage to ask for help than not to. I discuss this issue more in a later chapter titled *Dealing With People* on page 48.

Besides, asking for help will allow your family and friends to experience the joy of helping you. Taking care of Chris was one of the highlights of my life; if she had tried to do everything herself she would have denied me that satisfaction in addition to creating more stress on herself. All of our friends loved helping; it made them feel good.

2. You may not be able to make proper decisions regarding your own care. It's frightening to be diagnosed with a serious illness and you are likely to be confused, worried, and in shock. As a result, you may not be thinking clearly or objectively and your treatment decisions could very well be compromised.

3. If you refuse to discuss and share your treatment with your family and friends, they will be left with nothing but fear and despair. You may think that you are saving them from additional stress and worry by not "scaring" them with the details but, in fact, you will be making it worse for them. The more they are included, the more they will know, and the more they know the less fear and stress they will feel.

"... it is vitally important that you discuss these 'permissions' out loud, in advance"

Chris's brother lives 450 miles away; naturally he was terribly worried and felt helpless because he was so far away. Chris and I were very forthcoming when it came to the details of her condition and treatment, and he told us that he found it comforting to be kept in the loop. The same was true for Georgia, Chris's sister, who came to every appointment she possibly could. By staying involved it was not only comforting to Chris, but it was comforting for Georgia. How would *you* feel if someone important to you was very sick and they didn't include *you*?

4. Sharing your fears helps reduce them. It's a funny thing about human nature; the more you talk about what you're afraid of, the less afraid you will be. And here's an added bonus: sharing your feelings draws you closer to the person with whom you share them.

Permission to be sick. Another very important permission you must give the patient, and the patient must give herself, is the permission to be sick. It is nobody's fault, so neither of you should spend any time trying to fix the blame on her for getting sick because she didn't do this or she should have done that; it just doesn't matter. The only thing that matters is that you a), remove as much stress as possible b), get the proper treatment, and c), get that treatment without delay. Also, by giving herself permission to be sick, the patient has opened the door to dealing with it and can avoid denial, which can lead to delay of treatment and the serious consequences that are sure to follow.

Permission to make mistakes. You must also give each other permission to make mistakes along the way. I recognized immediately that if I was doing a lot of Chris's normal tasks around the house that I wouldn't necessarily do them exactly the way she would have. She had to cut me some slack on that, and when we discussed it she agreed. On the other hand, she knew that even though she would try to be nice to me, she would probably snap at me when she wasn't feeling well. She had to know that it was okay with me and that I would understand.

Permission to be afraid. Last but not least, you must give each other permission to be afraid. These are scary times, and you will both feel more comfortable if you know that the other will understand.

Communication is the key, and it is vitally important that you discuss these "permissions" out loud, and in advance. Set ground rules for what is and isn't okay to say, do, and share with others. This is your illness and you obviously can function in any way that is acceptable to both of you, but you must discuss the situation in advance so that you both know what "acceptable" is in your scenario, *before* it becomes a problem.

April 24:
The Surgeon

We actually arrived at Dr. Loman's office a little early and, right off the bat, got a nice surprise: Georgia, Chris's sister, was in the waiting room! Due to busy lives, Chris and Georgia hadn't seen too much of each other the previous few years so this was great. Georgia, who has been a teacher for almost 35 years near Los Angeles, arranged for a substitute to take her class for the day so she could be there for this important appointment. It was the first of many times that she would show her support by rearranging her life in order to be there for her little sister.

Dr. Loman examined Chris and looked at the seven-month-old mammograms I had brought. We were amazed to hear him say that, even though he knew the lump was there and exactly where it was, he couldn't see it on those films! He went on to say that, judging from the size of the lump, it had been growing there for as long as eight years! Why didn't it show on the mammogram? Why hadn't she been able to feel it before now? Good questions for which he had no good answer. As it turned out, no one else would be able to answer those questions either.

Dr. Loman felt that the best course of action would be a "lumpectomy with sentinel node biopsy." More medical mumbo jumbo; I will attempt to explain it even though I am not a doctor (and don't play one on TV). A "lumpectomy" is a surgical procedure in which the lump is removed from her breast along with a very small amount of good tissue surrounding the tumor, leaving everything else intact. In doing so the doctor is looking for "clean margins," which means that the removed tumor is completely surrounded by healthy tissue, indicating that they got all of it.

Naturally, the biggest concern is whether the cancer has spread to other parts of the body, which happens as a result of cancerous cells traveling through the lymph system (which is sort of like the body's "sewer system"). The lymph system receives drainage from various parts of the body and this drainage is pumped along through the system by the lymph nodes. If the lymph nodes contained cancerous cells, then it was likely that cancer cells had entered the lymph system and there was a higher risk that the cancer was growing elsewhere.

The trick here was to remove as few lymph nodes as possible in order to make this determination, which is where the "sentinel node biopsy" comes in. They would look at the first lymph node (the "sentinel" node) that receives drainage from the breast to see if it is involved with cancer. If it was *not* involved, then there is a 99% chance that the cancer was limited to the breast and had not spread. If it *was* involved, they would remove more lymph nodes to get a better idea of how many were involved, which would give them a better idea how likely it was that the cancer had spread. The purpose, then, of identifying and removing only the sentinel node was to be able to avoid removing more lymph nodes than necessary.

But how would they know which lymph node was the sentinel node? They are very clever: a few hours before the surgery, a radioactive dye would be injected into the lump. It, along with normal fluids, would drain into the lymph system and the dye could be followed with some sort of expensive machine (my own 'medical' term!) that would show the first node that received the dye. That, ladies and gentlemen, is the sentinel node. During surgery, guided by the image from the radioactive dye, they would remove the sentinel node and, while Chris was on the table, determine whether it contained cancerous cells. If it *did,* additional nodes would be removed for later biopsy. If not, they could be fairly certain that the cancer had not entered the body through the lymph nodes.

The bottom line was that the sentinel node biopsy would minimize the number of nodes that they removed, and allow whatever had to be done to be done in a single surgery.

Dr. Loman's surgical scheduling nurse said she would schedule the procedure as soon as possible, but that it would take a while because so many different departments were involved. Naturally, we wanted it done as soon as possible.

Dealing with People

After the diagnosis, it quickly became evident that there was another aspect of this situation that neither of us had anticipated: dealing with other people and their reactions to the news that Chris had cancer.

Chris and I enjoy the solitude and privacy that the mountains provide. We spend most of our time together and even though we see friends from time to time, we feel content being by ourselves. However, after Chris's diagnosis with breast cancer, we quickly realized that many people would want to be and would have to be included in our crisis. Our solitude and privacy were to disappear for a while; which we realized quickly when we returned home from one of the first appointments to find 21 messages on our answering machine!

In trying to include all those that cared about Chris in her care and in the progress she was making, I tried to create a balance that would give both us and those that cared about us some peace.

Everyone is different and everyone deals with a serious illness in his or her own way. For example, some people reacted to our news by telling us a story about a friend or relative who had had breast cancer. *Sometimes the story was even about someone who died from breast cancer.* We would gasp (to ourselves) at what we were hearing. What were they thinking? Why would they tell us such a thing? I'm sure they didn't realize the impact such a story might have on us, but rather they somehow wanted to let us know that they *thought* that they had some understanding of our situation. It was important for us to realize the reasons for the stories, and it was important that we quickly learned how to deflect that kind of conversation when we heard it coming.

There were also the people who wanted to help. And, because they were trying to deal with their own concerns and fears, it really came across that they *needed* to help. Their need was so strong, in fact, that it became difficult for me to deal with them. An offer to help came across more like a *demand* to help, which caused me to feel enormous pressure, especially if I didn't need or want what they were offering. I was using almost everything I had to keep Chris and myself going, and I just didn't have the energy to think of ways that individual people could help us, or to accept things that I didn't want or need just to meet *their* needs.

One solution was to say, "Please make us some meals; we don't have time to cook." Many of them did, and it was wonderful! Another solution was to use humor. If, for example, a female friend said, "If there's *anything* I can do, *please* let me know. I'll do *anything*. Really. *Anything*." I would respond with something like, "Well, I *have* been pretty lonely lately..." They knew I wasn't serious, but it got a laugh and usually (but not always) diffused the stress of finding something for them to do.

Another pressure we faced was returning all of the concerned phone calls from family and friends. Given our relative solitude, you can imagine the stress of a sudden onslaught of caring, concerned people who wanted to know how Chris was doing. After word of Chris's diagnosis spread around our small mountain community, it was immediate and it was amazing.

What to do? Under the best of circumstances, I spend little time on the phone and yet now I was faced with the tedious prospect of telling the same stories over and over. I thought it was wonderful that so many people cared enough to ask and I certainly wanted to share what was going on, but I just didn't have the time or energy to do it. My solution was twofold.

First, Kate, my assistant, returned as many calls as she could on my behalf. When people asked if there was anything they could do to help, she would tell them to bring food when Chris was recovering from surgeries. This helped me a great

> **" . . . the *very best* thing I did to keep people informed was to communicate by email."**

deal because it took away the burden of shopping for food and preparing meals when Chris needed the most help. Kate even coordinated who would bring what and when in order to even-out the flow. She is pretty ingenious.

The other thing that I did, the *very best* thing that I did to keep people informed was to communicate by email. Being basically a computer geek, it was easy for me to put together an email list and send one message to everyone on the list. Nearly everyone that was interested in Chris's progress had an email address, so it was the perfect solution. I wrote extensive updates every couple of weeks and sent them to everyone on the list. Our friends were informed, I gave the information just once, I went into much more detail than I would have on the phone, I could write when it was convenient for me (often very early in the morning), and we had a permanent record. I even created a page on my website containing all of the updates; each new update referred to that page, so anyone could get caught up on past messages no matter when they were added to the list. Plus, I posted some photos on the website when appropriate, so I could share those as well. And, best of all, our friends loved it!

__Note:__ you, too, can communicate with your family and friends by email by using The Patient/Partner Project website, which I developed for that very purpose. There you can create a private email list and then post progress reports. Whenever you post a report, everyone on your private list gets an email inviting them to read what you've written. It is easier to use this service than to create your own private list because 1), all of your messages are archived and can be read at any time when someone wants to "catch up" and 2), people can sign themselves up *to receive your notices without you having to add them to your list. The system is completely private because no one can read your reports unless they know the unique Member ID that you selected when you registered. Best of all, this service is free! Check it out at www.ThePatientPartnerProject.org (You can see all of the messages that I sent by going to the website and viewing messages for Member ID "EXAMPLE")*

The outpouring of love and caring was astounding and, frankly, caught us by surprise. There was even a note in our P.O. box from our postmistress to come to the counter, where she presented Chris with a plant in a cute, multi-colored ceramic teapot! The biggest surprise, though, was the reaction of the subscribers to my "Big Bucks in a Bathrobe" newsletter for small businesses. The tone of the newsletter has always been informal and personal, and my subscribers seem to enjoy that. Each issue features a short story about something that happened on the ranch, so my readers feel that they know Chris and our animals. Many have even written to say how much they enjoy getting a glimpse into our lives. About a month after the diagnosis I ran an article in the newsletter called "Priorities" in which I talked about Chris's condition and how it changed all of my priorities. It had been the first mention of Chris's illness. Here it is:

Priorities
by Dave Balch, "The Stay-at-Home CEO™"

Unfortunately, most of us need a little reminder every now and then about what is really important. Something will happen in our lives and we just sort of sit up, slap our foreheads stupidly, and say "DOH! Of course! I knew that, but I forgot that I knew that!"

The trouble is that we never know when that's going to happen and, when it does, it may be too late. If you lose a loved one in a tragic accident, how will you be able to say those things to them that you meant to say but never did?

My guess is that you probably don't have to think very hard to figure out your top priorities in life. Are you taking the time, however short, to think about it? And are you acting accordingly, spending your time and financial resources where it matters the most?

I just got a reminder of my own; my bride of 19 years was diagnosed with breast cancer. After we got the news I felt two profound emotions: fear and gratitude. The fear, of course, was about what the future held. The gratitude was for all the time we have been able to spend together by working at home for over 20 years.

After her first surgery we learned that the cancer had spread. When the situation is dire, it's easy to drop the things that used to be soooooooo important and focus on the things that really are.

I was in the parking lot of a local market and I saw a man and woman arguing about something. I thought about how their anger was probably over something that, in reality, just didn't matter a hoot. Someday they, too, may get a sudden reminder and they will hopefully realize how unimportant and insignificant those types of arguments usually are.

In going back over this article, it reads sort of negative, doesn't it? (SORT OF???) I don't mean to put you on a downer, I just want to suggest that you keep balance and perspective in your life. I want my reminder to serve as your reminder. It's amazing how quickly 'important' things can become unimportant.

It's easy to work a lot when you own a small business (I'll bet you didn't know that...), which makes it hard to achieve that balance and perspective without some conscious effort. Are your priorities in order? Don't wait for that giant reminder to come and slap you in the face. The next time you get angry with a loved one, ask yourself if it really matters that much.

One of my favorite movie quotes is from "Mr. Mom", one of Michael Keaton's first movies. In it, he loses his corporate job, can't find another, and his wife (played by Terri Garr) ends up going back to work for an advertising firm leaving him at home to take care of the kids. She ends up working too much, so he says these eight words to her.

Now I'm saying them to you:

"It's easy to forget what's important. So don't."

Within 24 hours of sending that issue, over 100 subscribers took the time to send an email to wish us well and tell me that Chris was in their prayers! These were complete strangers; I was blown away. I replied to each and every one of them, saying how much I appreciated that they took the time and that I felt like I had a new family. It was really very touching. As of this writing, over 350 messages of concern and encouragement have been sent by my subscribers. One of them even asked about Chris's hat size and favorite colors, then sent three hats that her daughters had made!

The bottom line is that interacting with interested and concerned people just goes with the territory. They truly care so, in my view, it is important to include them. On the other hand, it is difficult to keep everyone informed to their satisfaction. My advice: either get someone else to help you, create an email list and send them periodic updates yourself, or do it electronically at **www.ThePatientPartnerProject.org** where you can post private messages concerning your patient's progress and distribute access instructions to anyone who is interested. No one will be able to see your postings

"... interacting with interested and concerned people just goes with the territory."

unless they have the instructions from you, so your reports will be private among only those with whom you choose to share. This is a free service that I'm happy to provide for cancer patients and their partners.

Finally, I'd like to share a couple of stories to illustrate a few of the interactions we had with well-meaning people and to help prepare you for similar situations. Sometimes people feel that they need to give you advice or tell you "what is going to happen" based on their own experience or on the experiences of someone they know. *It is important to remember that no two cancer situations are exactly the same, and that no one else's experience will necessarily be indicative of your own.*

There was a woman who called to "counsel" us right after the diagnosis. We didn't know anything about anything at that time, and Chris wasn't afraid; we were just trying to sort it all out. This woman had had breast cancer five years earlier and considered herself an authority on the subject. She proceeded to tell us exactly what treatments Chris would be going through, which parts would be difficult and which parts would be *more* difficult, etc. She was obviously more interested in being dramatic and impressing us with how much she knew than in helping us. All she succeeded in doing, though, was make me mad. Here was someone who didn't know anything about our situation (and, by the way, didn't even ask) telling us what the course of treatment would be *(based on five-year-old medical technology)* and putting all sorts of frightening things into Chris's head. What was she thinking? When she hung up, Chris was laughing about it but I was storming around the house ready to kill. How was I going to be able to protect Chris from these well-meaning but insensitive people??

Another example of this occurred in a local restaurant after Chris's first chemotherapy treatment. A friend stopped at our table to say hello and introduced us to "Marlene," a friend of hers that was visiting from the city. When Marlene found

> **"It is important to remember that no two cancer situations are exactly the same, and that no one else's experience will necessarily be indicative of your own."**

out that Chris had breast cancer, she proceeded to tell Chris what would be happening to her. "Chemo isn't too bad except for the third one, that was the killer. Watch out for your third chemo; it's the worst."

I was *furious*. I wanted to leap across the table and strangle her. Why put negative expectations in Chris's head? (Chris had just finished her first chemo at the time.) How does she know what Chris is going to go through: she doesn't know a single thing about Chris or her condition!! How dare she give Chris something *else* to worry about?

I was livid. "It was the worst for *you*," I told her with a glare intended to kill. "Just because it was the worst for *you* doesn't mean it will be the worst for *her*." I tried to be civil but I guess I wasn't, because after she left Chris looked at me in amazement. She couldn't believe that her normally-passive Dave had been borderline rude to this woman. Once again, here was a well-meaning woman that just wasn't thinking about what she was saying. I'm sure that she meant no harm; it was just so *unnecessary* and so *insensitive*. I guess it was the part of me that was trying so hard to protect Chris that got so riled up. And, to top it off, I found out later that Marlene had had chemo *every week* (Chris's chemo was once every three weeks), thus making her statement even more off-the-mark and irrelevant for Chris's situation. It made me angry all over again.

There are two sides to this coin, however. One evening we met Becci Ripson, a woman with four children who was sitting at a table next to us in, coincidentally, the same restaurant where I almost strangled Marlene. (It was a different evening, however.) She accidentally overheard us talking with our friends about Chris's situation and she came over, introduced herself, and proceeded to ask some questions about Chris's condition and treatment. As we told her she listened, asked more questions, nodded her head in understanding, and made all the right noises.

"I went through all this about two years ago. Some of it was hard, but now I'm just fine. You will be too," she told us sweetly. "My hair came back with a vengeance; look how curly it is! It was never curly before, and I just love it!" She proceeded to tell us about all of the support she had during her treatment and how wonderful her life was now. "It's all just a bad memory," she continued. "You won't believe how quickly you forget the bad stuff."

I wanted to leap across the table at her, too, not to strangle her but to give her a hug! What a sweet, caring, and considerate person she was to offer-up such positive imagery. I told her how refreshing it was to hear someone share her experience without telling us something negative or scary. She agreed.

"People used to start telling me stories about someone they knew and I would cut them off mid-sentence, telling them, 'If this has an unhappy ending stop right now: I don't want to hear it.'" She was all smiles and the positive energy just oozed out of every pore. She was wonderful.

Why am I telling you all of this? Two reasons.

First, I'm hoping to create a new awareness of the kinds of things people *shouldn't* say when they discover someone has cancer. Chris's theory is that when most people hear this kind of news they feel that they have to say *some*thing but they don't know what, so they say the first thing they can think of that is even remotely related. It may be inappropriate, but at least it's *something* and it comes out before it can be edited. As we have seen, this can get us into trouble. My opinion is that the best thing you can do is to show interest by asking questions and expressing concern and, perhaps, a willingness to help. But remember not to become a burden by *insisting* that you be allowed to help.

The other reason for this section was to prepare you for the inevitable: dealing with friends, family, and well-meaning people who know (or think they know) what you are going through. There is no escaping it; dealing with other people is part of the job description. Perhaps, by being forewarned, you can handle the rough spots better than I did; I found that I had little tolerance for inconsiderate things that were said. Chris, though, knew that they meant well and gave them a huge break.

April 29:
The First Second Opinion

You have to take responsibility for your own care. As I write this, there is a story in the news about a woman who was diagnosed with breast cancer and had a double mastectomy (*both* breasts were removed), only to find out that the hospital had made a mistake in the lab results and she didn't have cancer after all. This is a tragic, horrific story that could probably have been prevented had they gotten a second opinion.

The cancer diagnosis is pretty scary. The days and weeks immediately after it is handed down are not the time to go hide in a corner; the patient and partner must take an aggressive stance and do everything they can to not only ensure that they get the *best* care, but that they get the *appropriate* care as well. The patient will pay the ultimate price for improper care, so it ends up being their own responsibility to make sure that that doesn't happen.

In our case, Chris was overwhelmed and in somewhat of a state of shock by the situation and couldn't really think clearly or objectively enough to make the calls and arrange the appointments. I, too, was inclined to just go along with the program. Thank heavens for our friend, Anne.

I had a conversation with Anne, a very close friend who happens to have a consulting practice in the medical field. Forcefully and persistently, yet politely (!) she "encouraged" me to get a second opinion. I knew she was right, but was so overwhelmed with what was going on that I just couldn't bring myself to make all of the calls. Who would I call? What would I say? What if I offended Dr. Loman? What if the second opinion was different? *Then* what would I do?

"Forcefully and persistently, yet politely, she 'encouraged' me to get a second opinion."

My stress level was soaring. I hit the phones and ended up spending almost six hours making calls and researching on the Internet. Being a basically positive person and trying to "think big" as much as possible, I decided to try for the very best breast cancer treatment center in Southern California regardless of where it was. Living in the mountains and not being particularly close to anything, I knew that there would be a lot of driving involved no matter what we did. Just staying with Dr. Loman involved 75 miles (90 minutes) each way for every treatment and appointment, so the location of the second opinion really didn't matter in the grand scale of things. Besides, how could I, in good conscience, compromise Chris's treatment in the name of convenience? Simple answer: I couldn't.

I called many people trying to get recommendations, including Anne who contacted some of her clients to see what they knew. It soon became clear that one of the best places to go would be the Revlon/UCLA Breast Center at The University of California, Los Angeles (UCLA). Even though I knew it was about 100 miles through downtown Los Angeles (about 2 hours' drive each way with no traffic, and there's never "no traffic"), I figured that the only thing that mattered was that Chris got the best care no matter what.

When I called UCLA, the person I needed to speak to wasn't there so I left a message and hoped that they would call back promptly. While I was waiting, I called five other highly recommended institutions to see if and when they could see Chris. In the process of doing this, and waiting for UCLA to call back, I made appointments at four of them, ranging from 10 days to two weeks out. This, too, was a major cause for stress because I needed to go to the Book Expo in New York City the following week for a book that I was promoting for my "Stay-at-Home CEO" business; that trip would have to be cancelled in order to keep any of these appointments

Thankfully, UCLA called me back and I was able to make an appointment for the following Monday at noon with Dr. Mai N. Brooks, a Surgical Oncologist. Perfect! We were thrilled! Not only did we get into the institution that was our first choice, we only had to wait two business days and I could probably still go to the Book Expo in New York (again, depending on the surgery date)!

The next day I called to cancel all of the appointments I had made while waiting for UCLA to call me back. Then I called some friends who were connected to the Los Angeles medical scene to see if they had heard of Dr. Brooks. They asked around and found that she was not only well known and well regarded in the medical community, but that she was also "very kind and caring." I felt so much better that we were doing the right thing and getting the best advice possible.

My trip to New York for the Book Expo was a major concern during all of this scheduling. With the lucky appointment at UCLA, it was apparent that I could still go, assuming that the surgery was scheduled for a date after I returned. It was important to me to go to the Expo because I had just created an electronic book ("eBook") titled "Confessions of the Stay-at-Home CEO" and I needed to attend several seminars and meet with several people in the book business in order to figure out what to do next. The pressure was on because I had a

---

"... the patient and partner must take an aggressive stance and do everything they can to not only ensure that they get the *best* care, but that they get the *appropriate* care as well."

"... juggling my life was becoming my way of life."

number of things to get ready before I left, including a demo CD-ROM containing samples of my book, speaking videos, sample newsletters, etc. Since this was my first CD, there was a considerable learning curve as I researched various software and methods of doing what I needed to do. Then, of course, there was the doing! If the surgery was scheduled during the time I would be gone, I would cancel the trip and the Book Expo would just have to get along without me. I certainly hoped it wouldn't play out that way, but I was prepared. I was learning that juggling my life was becoming my way of life.

Now it's time for you to meet Gail and Sonia, our dear friends on the mountain who live down the street from our first home up here. We have known them and been close for 14 years now. They are both psychoanalysts; Sonia retired a few years ago but Gail is still in practice in Los Angeles. She has a second home in the city in which she has an office where she sees patients Monday through Thursday. They are wonderful to us and incredibly generous; we feel like they are family. Hmmm... considering all the jokes about crazy families, let me say that they're *better* than family!! Gail has generously let me use her Los Angeles home to spend the night on various occasions when I had to be in the city early the next morning. And, by happy coincidence, that home is only 2 miles from UCLA!

It was now Thursday, April 25 and Chris had her appointment for the second opinion with UCLA's Dr. Brooks on the upcoming Monday. Being able to schedule a second opinion so quickly did, however, present a new problem because UCLA wanted to see the original biopsy slides which were still at a hospital at the bottom of our mountain.

It just so happened that I was going to a book fair at UCLA that weekend, the weekend before our UCLA appointment on Monday (what are the odds??), and I was planning to stay at Gail's house both Friday and Saturday nights. Maybe I could get lucky and be able to pick up the slides on my way to Los Angeles the next night. It was now too late to call the pathology lab to make arrangements but I would do so first thing the next morning.

It is truly amazing how something as seemingly simple as picking up pathology slides could become so complicated. And stressful. Early Friday morning I contacted the hospital where the biopsy had been performed. "Susie" informed me that the lab normally needed two days to retrieve slides. In addition, the lab was only open until 5:00 p.m. for pickups.

Now I was presented with two problems: first, I'd be lucky if the hospital could produce the slides that day and second, even if it did, the lab would close before I'd be able to get down the mountain to pick them up.

I tried to stay calm and explained the necessity of the situation, and Susie told me that they could 'probably' (gee, thanks a lot) get the slides before closing. That was great; now how could I pick them up after 5:00 so I could get them on my way into Los Angeles that night?

As it turned out, the hospital had a lab that's open 24 hours a day and Susie promised that the slides would be left there and I could pick them up any time. Perfect!

I called Susie at 4:30 that afternoon just to confirm that someone had, in fact, retrieved the slides and that they would be waiting for me in the 24-hour lab. It's a big hospital and I know how things can go wrong; I didn't want to show up at 8:00 that night and discover that someone goofed and the slides weren't there! After all, this was the only chance to get them before seeing Dr. Brooks, so it all had to work out.

And it did. I showed up at 8:00 p.m. and the slides were there. Whew!

Chris rode to Los Angeles with Gail on Sunday night (I had made arrangements for Kate to housesit) and we took Gail out for dinner at her favorite Japanese restaurant. We spent the night and, voila, we were right there for our appointment the next day at the Revlon/UCLA Breast Center with Dr. Brooks.

To say we were impressed with the Revlon facility would be a gross understatement. As soon as we walked in, we knew that we were in a special place because there was very little about the Center that felt 'medical'. Oh, sure, there were people walking around in white coats, and obvious medical equipment here and there, but that's where it ended. The walls in the examination rooms and in the halls were all rich, wood paneling. The shapes in the area were pleasing to the eye, not the usual cold, sterile, efficient-looking white hallways. The lighting was subdued, the floors were slate and marble, and there was artwork everywhere; beautifully framed paintings, sculptures on pedestals; it was obviously finished by talented, sensitive designers and it was, in a word, soothing. It was just the right place for stressed-out cancer patients and their stressed-out partners.

We waited less than five minutes until we were shown to an examining room, then waited less than five more minutes when Dr. Brooks walked in. She was tiny (even smaller than Dr. Win) and looked like she was about 15! We liked her before she said a word; there was an unmistakable aura about her that was very reassuring. We had agreed in advance not to tell her Dr. Loman's recommended treatment; we didn't want to put any ideas in her mind. We just wanted to hear her diagnosis, prognosis, and recommendations.

The best thing about Dr. Brooks was that she didn't seem rushed. I don't know about you, but I always feel uncomfortable seeing a doctor that seems like he/she can't wait to get to the next patient. Dr. Brooks walked in, sat down, crossed her legs, and said, essentially, "Tell me everything." She listened intently and asked many questions, which told me that she was not only listening to what Chris was saying but *hearing* it as well.

She examined Chris thoroughly, even more thoroughly than Dr. Loman had. She even "milked" the affected breast, obtaining some magic substance that she smeared onto a slide. (I offered her an imaginary three-legged stool for the milking, but she smiled and politely declined!) She, too, looked at the mammograms and could not see the lump, even though we all knew it had to have been there.

Dr. Brooks left the room, taking the slides with her, at which time Chris and I excitedly talked about how much we liked her. It was the first time we had been able to talk privately since we met her, and we were equally impressed with this lady. About ten minutes later Dr. Brooks returned and said that her recommendation would be to do a lumpectomy with a sentinel node biopsy; exactly the same procedure that Dr. Loman had recommended!

Then we asked the question: why, with no family history of breast cancer, would Chris get this? She told us that family history doesn't seem to be any indication of a tendency to get breast cancer, and that it is actually more common to see breast cancer patients with no family history of cancer. Go figure.

We were relieved to know that we were on the right track, and that one of the best breast care centers in the country concurred with the first recommended procedure. As scary as the surgery was, it suddenly didn't seem quite so scary. Just to be thorough, we left the slides from the biopsy so they could do a second opinion on that as well, but Dr. Brooks didn't expect the pathologist to find any differences in the diagnosis.

We had our second opinion in place and now we just had to wait for an actual surgery date to come from Dr. Loman's office. We pretty much knew what that day would be like: arrive at the hospital and check in, then to radiology where they will inject the radioactive dye into the lump, then wait about an hour, then into surgery, then recovery, then home. The big question, though, is what date and what time. In order to buy as much time as possible, I delayed my flight to New York from Tuesday morning to a redeye flight Tuesday night.

We got the call: the surgery was scheduled for May 10, about two weeks away. It was both scary and exciting at the same time; we both have always been very healthy and any surgery is way outside our comfort zone, but we also knew that we were doing absolutely the right thing. There is great comfort in knowing that you're on the right path, even if that path is a scary one.

Plus, the pressure was off because I knew I would be able to go to New York after all with no effect on the situation.

"There is great comfort in knowing that you're on the right path even if that path is a scary one."

May 1:
The New York Book Expo

I always enjoy visiting New York City, not only because I get to see my sister, but because I enjoy the hustle and bustle of the big city. For a few days at a time, that is: then I'm ready to head back to my peaceful life in the forest. The last time I had been there was six weeks after the terrorist attack on the World Trade Center, and I had had the privilege of working with the Red Cross, helping to feed the workers at the Mayor's Emergency Response Center. (If you would like to read the details of that experience, I have posted an extensive description of what it was like on the Internet at **www.CancerForTwo.com/redcross.htm**)

This was going to be a relatively inexpensive trip, which, considering our financial situation, was why I was able to go. I used frequent flyer miles to get there, I stayed with my sister who lives in a wonderful apartment that is ideally located and, as publisher of an Internet newsletter I got a free pass to the Book Expo.

Attending the Expo is always fun because I wear a bathrobe. Yes, you read that right: I wear a bathrobe because, as "The Stay-at-Home CEO" it is my trademark to do so. Two years earlier I had attended the Expo in Chicago and wore a white terrycloth robe everywhere I went. It was a big hit and everyone loved it. I was looking forward to this book event because it would be a nice break from the emotional roller coaster I had been on since Chris was diagnosed. What I didn't know was that attending the Expo was going to give me the opportunity to do something really special for Chris.

Book Expo America (BEA) is the largest show of its kind in the United States and is always held in late spring. It attracts thousands of publishers, book dealers, authors, and all manner of businesses related to the publishing industry. Publishers typically ask their most popular authors to sit for photos and to autograph copies of their latest books for those willing to stand in line. Some of the lines are short and some are *really* long, such as the lines for Al and Tipper Gore who were there to promote a new book.

In order to maintain some measure of crowd control, a limited number of tickets are handed out for signings and photo sessions on the day of those sessions. Tickets are free, but required if you want a photo with your favorite author or if you want to say hello and get a free, autographed copy of his/her book. While standing in line for a photo with an author that I am fond of, I overheard someone in line talking about Jean Auel, who was going to be there the next day. "I'm just dying to get her tickets," she said. "I'll be here at 7:00 a.m. tomorrow, you can bet on it!"

"*OH MY GOD!*" I thought to myself. "This is a golden opportunity to really surprise and thrill Chris." Chris had read Ms. Auel's first book, *"Clan of the Cave Bears,"* and every sequel as well and had recently mentioned that she couldn't wait for the next one in the series. The main character's name is "Ayla" and she has a horse and, well, that's all you really need to know about why Chris loves these books! Chris identifies strongly with Ayla and is certain that she was just like that in a previous life. Wouldn't it be a great surprise to bring home an autographed copy for Chris to read when she is recovering from surgery?? I knew right then and there that I simply *must* get this book for her.

The next morning I arrived at the Expo at 8:00 and the tickets for Jean Auel's book-signing *were already gone!* Aaaaahhh! There were tickets available for her photo session, however, so I grabbed one of those. While I was at the ticket kiosk I also got tickets for Al and Tipper Gore's book signing and photo session; two of each. Thinking positively, I figured I might be able to find someone with a Jean Auel book-signing ticket that would be willing to trade with me.

I then began to ask people at random if they had a Jean Auel ticket they would like to trade for an Al Gore ticket; I felt like I was 14 years old again and trading baseball cards! I got no bites, however, so I thought I'd ask Ms. Auel personally at the photo shoot if she could somehow get me into her autograph line.

There was a long line at the photo shoot but I knew I'd get in because I had a ticket. When I finally reached Ms. Auel, I said, "My wife absolutely *loves* your books and she has just been diagnosed with breast cancer. It would mean so much to both of us if I could get a copy of your new book for her to read while she's recovering from surgery, but I couldn't get a ticket for your autograph line. Is there any possible way you could get me in?"

She got a very sweet and concerned look on her face and she took my hand in hers. "There really isn't anything I can do, but if you can get a copy of the book I would be happy to sign it for you." She would be at BEA the next day, and she told me how to find her. "Please give your wife my regards and best wishes." Then she wrote a little note to Chris on the back of my photo-shoot ticket.

Not one to be easily discouraged, I got in the autograph line two hours later even though I didn't have a ticket. I wasn't sure if or how I would get through, but they hadn't checked tickets in several of the lines the day before, so maybe I'd get lucky. If not, I'd buy a copy of the book on my way home and have it autographed the next day. One way or the other, my Chris was going to have that book!

Suddenly I noticed a man working his way down the line collecting tickets. Oh, no! I tried to be inconspicuous, *standing there in my bathrobe (!)*. He tapped me on the shoulder to ask for my ticket, so I turned to him and said, "I don't have a ticket, but my wife has just been diagnosed with breast cancer and it would really mean a lot to her to have this book to read while she is recovering. Could you please let me through anyway?" Gulp. He was very nice and said, "Sure, go ahead, and I hope she gets better soon." I felt tears come to my eyes; I wanted to hug that nice man! Positive thinking and persistence paid off!

When I got to the table, Ms Auel recognized me and was happy to sign a copy of the book, which was about the size of a small house: over 700 pages! That will certainly give Chris many hours of escape from her situation. I was ecstatic.

When the BEA event was over, something fascinating happened: all of the books on display were given away! All I had to do was ask and they were happy to give them to me because it was so much easier than hauling them home. I had seen several books about horses that I knew Chris would like, so I picked them up for her as I left.

But my biggest prize, the one I knew she would be happiest about, and the one that I felt I had *earned*, was *"The Shelters of Stone"* by Jean Auel. I couldn't wait to see the look on Chris's face!

I wasn't disappointed. Naturally, I was too excited to wait until her chemotherapy started, so I gave her *"The Shelters of Stone"* immediately. Her face lit up and so did my heart. She was thrilled, saying, "I can't believe that it's out already" at least three times. When I told her the story about how I waited in lines and appealed to the kindness of the man who let me stay in line even without a ticket, she was very touched and gave me a big hug.

Was it worth the effort? YOU BET IT WAS!

May 10:
The Lumpectomy and Sentinel Node Biopsy

The surgery procedures were scheduled for 12:00 and 2:00; they would inject the radioactive dye into the lump at 12:00, and then remove the lump and sentinel node at 2:00. We were comfortable with the hospital because we had made a special trip there three days earlier (involving making arrangement for the animals and 90 minutes of driving each way) for Chris's pre-operative testing. After the tests were completed, we had familiarized ourselves with the locations of the various departments so we didn't have to worry about finding our way around; there was enough to think about.

Normal surgical instructions state that the patient should not have any food or water after midnight the night before surgery but, in this situation, that posed a serious problem for Chris because she tends to have hypoglycemic attacks caused by low blood sugar (she feels light-headed, flushed, and dizzy; sometimes even passing out) if she gets too hungry. So, one of my first orders of business when I returned from New York was to see if we could get the midnight stipulation changed.

As it turns out, the real requirement is that the patient not eat or drink anything 8 hours prior to surgery. Midnight is just the general rule, which makes it easier for them to request and easier for the patients to understand. I still had to jump through hoops, though, to get them to make an exception for us. As it turns out, they contacted the anesthesiologist and he told them about the 8-hour rule, so Chris had a "reprieve" until 6:00 a.m. That, she could handle. It just goes to show that

> **"It just goes to show that you shouldn't be afraid to question some of the rules; they may not be what they seem."**

you shouldn't be afraid to question some of the rules; they may not be what they seem.

After that issue was resolved, I had to make sure that everything was arranged for the night before the surgery. That meant making a hotel reservation, lining up Kate to housesit, and making plans with Ken for dinner. Plus, there was another issue: after the surgery how would Chris be able to let me know if she needed something when she couldn't get out of bed? Our house was too big for a "sick bell" and, besides, what if I was down at the barn or walking the dogs in the forest? The perfect solution: walkie-talkies! (These are sold as "Family Radios"; they can be found in just about any store that sells electronics and you can get a pair of them for anywhere from $50 to $200.) I knew that Kate had a pair of them that she and her husband used when they went skiing, so I arranged to borrow them. It was important to anticipate the things that would be needed in the days following the surgery; anything I could do in advance would make it that much easier when the time came.

The night before the surgery Chris and I went with Ken to a wonderful Japanese restaurant for dinner. Chris didn't seem too worried about the surgery, mainly because (I think) Ken had performed an outpatient surgery on her elbow a couple of years earlier so she felt like she knew the drill. ("Outpatient" means that the patient goes home the same day as the surgery.)

When dinner was over we went to the hotel, which was an experience in itself because, as it turned out, it was in a pretty seedy neighborhood. I was both surprised and disappointed because the hospital itself is in a nice area and we were only a few miles away. Had I known, I would have tried to find a different place.

At that point it didn't really matter, though, so we walked up the outside stairway past a few shady-looking characters who were sitting on the stairs about halfway up, went into our room, and locked the door securely. Safe!

At 5:00 the next morning I got up and drove a few blocks to Denny's to get Chris some coffee, oatmeal, and an English muffin. I brought it back to the room, awakened Chris, and discovered to my great dismay that it looked like there was about half as much oatmeal as there should have been. I drove back and they were more than happy to give me more, even though they had given me the proper amount to begin with.

Chris had her breakfast and finished up about 5:59, so we were right on target: no food or drink after 6:00 a.m. Then we both went back to sleep for a couple of hours.

Just before we left for the hospital we took one last 'before' photo of her breast... she didn't know how this would all play out and she wanted to be able to remember how she looked before everything started happening.

We got to the hospital right on time and there, sitting in the lobby, was Georgia! Bless her heart! We followed Chris into the surgical preparation area where she was assigned a bed (well, it was really a gurney) and she changed into her little surgical gown and they started the IV. The three of us were having a great conversation, laughing a lot and wreaking all manner of havoc when Ken showed up to take me to lunch. Chris would be going up for the dye injection soon and Georgia would stay with her until I got back from lunch. We were optimistic and confident that this procedure would be the end of it and life would soon return to normal.

Just a few minutes after I returned from lunch the anesthesiologist arrived and he was just about as pleasant and reassuring as he could be. He had been the first person on the list of recommendations from Ken, and I could see why. He injected something into the IV and I knew that Chris would soon be unaware of us, so I kissed her and wished her luck and told her that I would be there every second and would be at her side as soon as they let me.

Then the big moment came when they whisked her off to the operating room. We said our goodbyes and I told her I loved her. Through her fog, she looked up at Georgia and said, "Take care of Dave." Then she was gone and I was crying like a baby. And the wait began.

Georgia left to run some errands and would return shortly. A nurse had told me where the surgeon would look for me when it was over, and also said not to expect him for about 90 minutes. I had brought my computer to do some work, but just couldn't concentrate so I went for a walk and bought some food at a nearby mini-mart for Chris to eat on the way home. I remembered that she had fainted when we got home from her elbow surgery because she hadn't had enough to eat. I put the food in the car and then just hung around in the waiting room. The 90-minute mark came and went and I started to get worried. After 2 hours he appeared and I could tell from the look on his face that the news was not what I wanted to hear.

He characterized the situation as "difficult": he had cut out as much of the lump as he dared but the margins were not clean, so he cut some more and then cut again, but never got the clean margins that he was looking for. The bottom line: he could not remove the entire tumor so some of it was still in her breast.

The sentinel node was removed and analyzed and it *was* involved with cancer, so they removed additional lymph nodes under her arm, which were sent to the pathology lab for analysis.

All through this explanation I felt myself going into a sort-of trance, and in a strange way left my own body and observed the scene from another place, all the time hearing him but feeling as if I were watching someone else receive this news. My eyes teared-up as he was speaking and he looked like his might as well; he was obviously a very caring man who had done the best he could in a tough situation.

Damn! My fantasy had been that he would come out and say, "We got all of the tumor and it's in the trash where it belongs. The sentinel node was clean, so go home and have a nice life."

"What's next?" I asked him.

He said, "I'll see you next week and we'll have the lab report by then."

"When can I see her?"

"They will come and get you in about 30 minutes."

So I waited again, wondering how I was going to break the news to her. I had truly thought that this would be the end of it, once again falling victim to the "this-happens-to-other-people-not-us" mentality. His news was reality hitting me in the face and I knew that we were sailing off into uncharted waters.

When they called me I couldn't get into the recovery room fast enough. There she was with a sleepy, but concerned look on her face.

"I just saw Dr. Loman and he told me the news. What's going to happen to me?"

"The only thing you need to worry about right now is recovering from this surgery. The rest will happen when it happens." I sounded much braver than I felt.

That's when it really struck me how important it is to concentrate on the problem at hand and I came up with a phrase that would serve us well in the coming months: "don't go there 'til you get there."

Georgia returned and found her way to us. She, too, was stunned at the news but she understood the importance of staying positive and in the moment and we soon began laughing again.

Then the nurse came in to tell me about Chris's drain.

HER DRAIN?? My wife has a DRAIN? What the...

She removed a fold of Chris's gown and there was a rubber bulb, similar to the bulb at the end of a turkey baster, fastened to the gown with a safety pin. It was clear and it looked like it had been squeezed because it was collapsed on one side. One end of the bulb had a hole with a little cap, and the other end was attached to a clear flexible, rubber tube which disappeared under the gown and, presumably, into my bride. Inside the bulb was some pale red fluid.

"You need to empty this fluid twice a day into one of these little cups," the nurse told me, producing a stack of small paper cups about the size of the circle you can make with your thumb and index finger. "The cups have markers on the side that indicate the amount of fluid you've removed, and we need you to write down that measurement each time you empty it, then give those measurements to the doctor when you see him."

Uh-huh.

"To empty the drain you remove this little cap, point the end down into the cup, and squeeze the bulb. When it's empty, squeeze the bulb again so it is collapsed before putting the cap back on. The bulb, trying to expand back to its original shape, will apply suction to the drain, causing the fluid to run into the bulb."

She demonstrated and it wasn't really complicated; a little icky, but not complicated. (Although I've kidded you a little in this explanation, after picking up every bodily excretion you can imagine from the parrot, cats, dogs, and horses for many years, I'm not squeamish and didn't really have any trouble with the instructions or the prospect of doing this. It is fun, however, to pretend that it's a big deal because the reactions I get are priceless!)

We were also given a prescription for pain medication, so I left Chris and Georgia together and went to the pharmacy to fill it.

By 5:00 the hospital was ready to release her, so the nurse helped Chris get dressed and they took her out front in a wheel chair (standard operating procedure in any hospital whether you can make it on your own or not). She got into the car (gingerly!) and off we went to face the worst rush-hour traffic of the day.

Chris reclined the chairback and munched on the crackers that I had purchased earlier. We talked a little and she slept a lot, which is just what I was hoping she would do.

I used the carpool lane and we sailed past a lot of the traffic, but I was just sure that we would get pulled over by the Highway Patrol because, from outside the car, it looked like I was riding alone. (On many California freeways, the left lane is designated as a "carpool lane", restricted to vehicles with two or more occupants. The idea is to encourage people to ride together, thereby reducing the amount of traffic and pollution. If you are alone in the carpool lane, that's a big no-no.)

It might have just been my imagination, but I'm sure that I saw other drivers giving me dirty looks. I wondered what I should do if I saw those red lights in my rear-view mirror while in the carpool lane, but luckily didn't have to find out. I decided that the next time I had an opportunity, I would ask a police officer about it. After all, I'm not sure if the law stated that there must be two or more occupants *in* the vehicle, or two or more occupants *visible* in the vehicle. This was the first of many, many times that I would be in this situation.

I've always enjoyed driving, and on long drives I typically listen to audiotapes. Sometimes I choose motivational tapes; sometimes educational tapes pertaining to a topic relevant to something I'm working on. I just hate to waste the time when I could be learning something that would help me or my business. But I was under so much stress that I just couldn't handle it. The idea of having to actually *think* made me tighten up another notch. I tried listening to the news, but radio news wasn't any more tolerable than the television news I couldn't stand to watch. Even music stations were annoying to me because the stress had reduced my patience to zero, and I got very annoyed if I had to listen to a song that I didn't like. So we rode along in silence. I decided that the driving time would be my chance for some moments of peace, and it was wonderful.

Uh-oh. I suddenly realized that when we got home the dogs would be very happy to see us, jumping and hopping about with great enthusiasm. Obviously this would be a problem with fresh stitches and the drain, which was pinned with a safety pin to her clothing. What if one of the dogs accidentally hooked the tube of the drain on her paw and pulled it… aaaahh! I didn't even want to go there. I did, however, devise a plan.

It took over 2 hours to make the 90-minute drive home. When we finally got there, Chris stayed in the car while I closed the garage door and went into the house to greet the dogs. Then I let them out so they could run around and, hopefully, use up some of that pent-up energy while I went back into the garage to help Chris out of the car and into the house. (Our entire property is fenced, so there is no concern that they might run off.) Chris was seated with all sensitive areas carefully protected and she was ready for action when I let the dogs back into the house and they gleefully, but safely, greeted her.

I helped her into bed, made sure that her water and walkie-talkie were where she could reach them, and she went to sleep while I went about the evening chores of walking the dogs and feeding the horses, cats, dogs, and myself, all of which takes about 2 hours. After checking on her I went downstairs to my office and dealt with email and a host of business-related stuff, after which I had to shut down the house for the night.

"Shutting down the house" involves cleaning the parrot cage, cleaning the cat boxes, taking the dogs outside one last time, and cutting up carrots for the horses. Then I have to take the carrots down to the barn, check that the automatic pellet feeders are full of feed, check that their water is clean, and give the horses the carrots as well as some hay and a mixture of supplements. Another hour, minimum.

The point is that there is one heckava lot to do! Normally Chris and I share these chores but now that she was out of action I got to do it all, plus tend to her needs as well as my own and those of my business. It was the first of many late evenings for me.

By the time I got to bed around 1:00 am, I found myself feeling extremely depressed and discouraged. What was going to happen to Chris? How would I be able to pay for everything when I didn't have much time for work? I didn't even *feel* like working, and the projects I had been excited about held no interest for me any more. It all just seemed so hopeless. Above the din of all of those voices, I tried to remind myself that I was tired and everything seems worse when you're tired. I just forced it all, well most of it anyway, out of my mind and tried to go to sleep. Instead, I found myself crying tears of fear, frustration, and hopelessness.

In order not to bother Chris, I moved into one of the guest bedrooms but slept with the walkie-talkie on the pillow next to mine. That way, if she needed anything, I could jump up and run in there. The first night was quiet.

When I checked on her the next morning she was awake and very hungry so I whipped up some coffee, oatmeal, and an Australian toaster biscuit. I put it all on a tray and brought it in to her so she could sit up and eat in bed. It was just like my mother used to do for me when I was sick, and it felt good to take care of her that way.

After she ate, it was time to empty the drain. I got the little cup, opened the end of the drain, pointed it into the cup and squeezed. The sound of the fluid rushing into the cup freaked Chris out, so I immediately stopped squeezing.

"Let's sing," I suggested.

" . . . everything seems worse when you're tired."

> "With a little creativity, it is possible to turn something unpleasant into something fun."

"Good idea," she said. "How about 'Oh, Canada'?" (Many years ago we had seen a 12 year-old girl belt out a rousing version of "Oh, Canada", Canada's national anthem, on the David Letterman show. Ever since then, we've enjoyed singing it on occasion, trying to emulate that girl's bold style. Why she thought of that song at that moment is somewhat of a mystery, except that we always sing it in a fun setting for a fun reason, and that's just what we needed.)

So we started singing loudly together and I emptied the rest of the fluid into the cup without a problem. And we laughed about it. With a little creativity, it is possible to turn something unpleasant into something fun, a technique we would use many times in the coming months.

Chris wasn't supposed to get the dressings wet, so her shower became an event for both of us. Chris designed our shower so it would be easy to bathe the Saint Bernard we had at the time the house was built, so it is rather large and has a hand-held showerhead on the end of a 10-foot hose. Perfect for precise aiming of the spray. Since they had removed lymph nodes under her right arm she couldn't use that arm, so it was pretty much up to me to wash, rinse, and dry.

Soaping-her-up was fun for both of us as I pretended to enjoy it much more than I should have, and she held the showerhead to direct the spray out of the way. If I got too "fresh", she would spray me a little as a fun "warning", but there was never any tension or animosity, just lots of laughter. Every now and then she would turn a certain way and get a shot of pain, or I would accidentally bump or touch something that hurt her, but she knew I was doing the best I could. She would yelp and then we'd go back to laughing.

Then came the drying. In order to effectively dry the 'private areas' I would scrunch the towel up length-wise, place it

"... if you can put some fun into something it's no longer a chore."

between her legs with one end in front and one in back, and then move the towel back and forth in a sawing motion. But Chris insisted that I make a noise while I was "sawing" that sounded like "VVVVOOOO-tah, VVVVOOOO-tah VVVVOOOO-tah!" We did that for every shower and laughed every time. It just goes to show that if you can put some fun into something it's no longer a chore.

Washing her hair was a completely different animal. I couldn't do it in the shower because there was no way to rinse her head and keep her dressings dry, so we needed to do it in the kitchen sink. The problem with that was that, because of her surgery, she couldn't bend over the sink. The counter next to the sink is just barely long enough for her to lie on with her legs bent, but getting up there and into that position was nearly impossible to do without a lot of pain. But this was her *hair*, after all, so the pain was incidental and she toughed it out.

Once she got into position the job was fairly easy, although I did need some training. Don't use too much shampoo, only put the crème rinse on the ends, wash it out but not *all* out, etc. I'm a quick learner, though, and after the first time I was semi-professional.

Drying her hair was the next stop on the training circuit. Drying my own hair was one thing, but drying someone else's is not as easy as it looks. It's sort of like trying to judge right and left, or forward and backward while looking in a mirror. Don't put the dryer too close, use the round brush like this, wave the dryer back and forth so the hair (and scalp) doesn't burn, and so on. Unfortunately, I got to be *too* good at it and she began asking me to do it when she could do it herself! She told Dale, her hair stylist and our good friend, that his job was in jeopardy. (She was very proud to tell anyone who would listen that I could use a round brush to get the ends to curl under.)

Due to my new-found shampooing, drying, and styling skills, Chris began to call me "Mr. Dave."

The four days between the surgery and the post-operative appointment with the surgeon were very busy. The morning would start with feeding the cats, walking the dogs, feeding the horses, picking up the manure, and then feeding the dogs and fish. When Chris woke up, I would make her breakfast and my own, then do the dishes, uncover the parrot, change the papers at the bottom of the cage, change his water and make him an English muffin, and water the plants outside including Chris's flower garden. Then it was shower time, first myself, then Chris. Maybe I would have a chance to check my email (maybe not), and then it was time for lunch and more dishes, let the dogs out, give the horses something to eat and, perhaps, spend an hour or so in the office.

Around 4:00 it was time to walk the dogs, feed the horses, feed the dogs, make (or get) something for dinner, more dishes, etc. Maybe a little more time to work and then it was time to close up the house and put everyone to bed. Dealing with Chris was the easy part; she was in good spirits and we had fun. Besides, I just loved looking at her. All of the other stuff started to become a drag and I found myself sinking into despair at least once a day. It's no big surprise that the more tired I got the more likely it was that I would feel that heavy, hopeless feeling, and start to tear-up. I tried not to let Chris know how I was feeling because she had enough to worry about.

It wasn't just her illness and the unthinkable notion that I might lose her, because that just didn't seem possible. (There's that "that-only-happens-to-other-people-but-not-us" mentality again.) I think that a lot of my despair and stress was financial, not only because our finances were borderline before this started, but because I didn't have much time to pursue my new career and thereby improve the situation.

Earlier in the year I had made an unsuccessful effort to land some speaking engagements, but in retrospect it was a good thing that I hadn't because I would have probably had to cancel them in order to be there for Chris. But I did have a weekly column in the local newspaper that I had to keep up with, as well as my e-mail based newsletter that came out every other week. In addition, I was sending an article out into the Internet cosmos every week in the hopes that other newsletters and websites would use them, thereby giving me exposure and getting new subscribers to my own newsletter. And, to top it off, I had a guest spot on our local cable channel news program every other Friday. None of these activities produced any income, but I did them because I considered each to be an investment in the future and would lead to something bigger and profitable. The pressure to keep up with even this meager commitment as well as taking care of Chris and all of our animals was immense.

May 15:
The Post Op Appointment

We left two hours before our scheduled appointment with Dr. Loman; I drove so Chris could sleep. Once again I found myself in the carpool lane, watching my rearview mirror for the red lights of a Highway Patrol officer who would only be able to see one person in the car. We arrived on time and there, in the waiting room, was Georgia, who had once again made arrangements for someone to watch her class for the day.

The three of us were shown into one of the smallest examination rooms I've ever seen, and when the doctor arrived it was crowded and warm in there. The news he had for us was not good.

First of all, since the margins were not clean he said that Chris needed a mastectomy, which was not something that she wanted to hear. In addition, the pathology report showed that 13 lymph nodes had been removed, and that 6 of them were involved with cancer cells. This didn't mean too much to us until he said that the generally accepted rule was that chemotherapy and radiation would be given if more than 4 were involved.

Now we were faced with a mastectomy *and* chemotherapy *and* radiation. Chris had told me for a very long time that if she ever had to have a mastectomy that she wanted to have reconstruction, so we asked about that. Dr. Loman told us that they don't recommend reconstruction until after radiation and he told us a generalized timetable that put the reconstruction over a year away. Chris was not happy with this news, to say the least.

Here's how it would play out. The reconstruction involved the insertion of implants to simulate the breast that had been removed. The implants would collapse during radiation, so they could not be inserted until several months after radiation was finished. Since the skin is somewhat hardened by radiation, the procedure would begin with insertion of a "tissue expander" under the skin. This is an outpatient surgery, but a surgery nonetheless.

Then, every week for about six weeks, Chris would come in and they would inject something into the tissue expander that would make it, uh, expand, stretching the radiated tissue outward to make room for the implant.

After that, there would be another surgery where the tissue expander was removed and replaced with the implant, which could, theoretically, be rejected by the body. And, by the way, the implant would have to be replaced every 10 to 15 years.

Yikes!

Then Chris asked Dr. Loman the big question. "Am I going to die? Is this going to kill me? If so, how long do I have?"

My fantasy was that he would say something like, "Don't be silly! Your case isn't serious and I'm sure you'll be fine."

He didn't.

He got very serious and I could tell that he felt like he was on the spot, which he was.

"The five-year survival rate for someone in your situation is about 50 to 60 percent," he told her. I could tell he didn't want to say it, and he sort of choked it out.

Chris went pale. "You mean I only have about a 50-50 chance of *living for five years*??" she asked him incredulously, her jaw dropping in disbelief.

He told us that with her type of cancer and the stage that she was in and the fact that it had spread to the lymph system, studies show that survival rate.

It was at that moment that Chris began to go into hypoglycemic shock. We'll never know if it was brought on by the bad news or if she truly didn't have enough food in her system, but I suspect that the news had something to do with it.

She got very hot and began to get dizzy. We always have individual-serving-size packets of honey close at hand for just this type of situation, but for some reason I didn't have any in my pocket and we couldn't find any in her purse. Cursing myself for being so unprepared, I ran from the examination room to the car to get some while Georgia helped cool her down with some wet towels. When I returned, Chris was flat out on the table and *Dr. Loman had left the room!* Can you imagine? He said he'd be back when we got her back up! We laugh about it now, but I must say I was, uh, "disappointed" in the doctor; what kind of doctor leaves the room when a patient begins to faint?

I gave Chris the honey and she came out of it rather quickly, as she always does when this sort of thing happens. I went to tell the doctor that it was "safe" to come back into the room, and he appeared a few minutes later.

He said that he wanted to do a bone scan, a test that would show whether the cancer had spread to her bones, and had scheduled one for her the following Monday. Also, he would be taking her case to the tumor board which was also on Monday, and that he'd like to see her again Monday afternoon.

Then he took a look at the drain, which he didn't want to remove just yet. He proceeded to "milk" the drain, which means that he pinched and held the tube with his left hand where it entered Chris's body, and then pinched the tube with his right thumb and index finger and, while pinching, slid the thumb and index finger along the tube all the way to the bulb, thereby clearing the tube of some bits of dried blood that were impeding the flow into the bulb. Interesting.

We left Dr. Loman's office and went to the pharmacy next to the hospital to get more of Chris's pain medication. While we were waiting there, Chris was admiring some betta fish (also known as "Japanese fighting fish") that were on display. Each one was in a glass bowl, swimming among the roots of a Chinese Evergreen plant. Male betta fish will fight with each other if given the chance, so they swim alone.

Chris decided that she wanted one as a symbol for her own fight which she characterized as "the fight of her life," so she picked one that was bright red and named it "Winston" after Winston Churchill; Chris had always admired Churchill because he was such a fighter in his own right and because he loved horses. There is simply nothing quite like owning a fighting fish named after a determined world leader to represent the fight of a lifetime.

We got the medication and left for Wal-Mart. Chris discovered that Georgia had never been to a Wal-Mart and, since Chris just loves Wal-Mart, she wanted to introduce her to its many delights. They had a grand time looking at everything. They were amazed to find lipsticks that would stay on for four days, and Georgia encouraged Chris to put a few of them on her arm to see how they looked with her coloring. (I guess this is something that women do; personally I've never shopped for lipstick.) When Chris tried to rub them off she discovered that they truly were four-day lipsticks: they wouldn't come off of her arm! They laughed and they laughed... and Chris had the marks on her arm for four days.

On the way home, Chris was sleeping in the back of the truck as she often did. We were driving along in the carpool lane and I heard Chris start to cry. Softly at first, it was the first (and only) time that I heard her cry about her illness. In a heart-wrenching tone that I had never heard come out of her, she choked out the words, "I don't want to die. Why is this happening to me?" and continued to sob.

It absolutely broke my heart. I couldn't hold or comfort her; I couldn't even touch her because she was in the back seat. My eyes teared-up and I had to concentrate on driving, but I knew that I had to say *something*. Or did I? Everything that I considered saying seemed hollow, empty, or just plain stupid. I was dying inside, not only at hearing her so distressed, but also at the thought that she might die.

What could I possibly say? I couldn't tell her not to cry; who am I to tell her not to cry or not to feel the way she did? She *needed* to cry. I couldn't tell her it would be okay, because I didn't know that and she knew that I didn't know that. I always feel that when something is wrong it is my responsibility to fix it; it's just a knee-jerk reaction that I have in many situations. I knew that I couldn't fix this, so I didn't say anything and just listened to her cry. It was one of the hardest things I've ever done, but I'm convinced it was the best thing I could have done under the circumstances. Sometimes the best thing you can do to help is to do nothing at all.

It seemed like she was crying for an eternity even though it was really only a few minutes; I will never forget those few minutes as long as I live.

"Sometimes the best thing you can do to help is to do nothing at all."

May 17:
The Second Second Opinion

After the bad news from Dr. Loman about Chris's survival chances, I did some scrambling to get back to UCLA for another second opinion. Not only did we want to know if Dr. Brooks concurred with the dreaded mastectomy recommendation, but we wanted to know her thoughts on Chris's chances of survival.

Once again, we were pleasantly surprised at how quickly Dr. Brooks could see us; in only two days, and in the middle of the day, too, which made it so much easier for us considering the two-hour drive to get there. She did, however, want to see the slides from the lumpectomy, so I made arrangements to pick them up on the way to UCLA; it was only about 20 miles out of the way.

As usual, Kate came to the rescue and worked on Monday to take care of the animals and, as usual, I drove while Chris slept in the back. I still couldn't handle listening to tapes, news, or music, so I just enjoyed the solitude.

When Dr. Brooks walked into the room we both felt better just seeing her; that unmistakable aura had once again come into the room with her. She admired Dr. Loman's work; the incision he had made was perfectly aligned with Chris's areola and would have been virtually undetectable when it healed except, of course, that the mastectomy would now make that irrelevant. It was, regardless, an outstanding job.

Dr. Brooks and Chris and I talked for a while. Dr. Brooks said that, assuming UCLA's pathology report was in agreement, she agreed that a mastectomy was indicated.

Chris asked about her chances for survival, and told Dr. Brooks that Dr. Loman had mentioned 50 to 60 percent. Dr. Brooks said that she thought it was more like 70 to 80 percent, and that we had to remember that, since "five-year survival rates" are the number of people who have survived at least five years, those people were treated using five-year-old technology. It stands to reason that people treated today will fare better than those treated five years ago due to refined procedures and medications, so the percentage of survivors is probably even higher than that. Besides, she said, that rate takes *all* patients into account, and Chris was younger than many and in better health than most to begin with, two facts that increased her percentages even more.

Isn't Dr. Brooks wonderful?

What about chemotherapy? Will Chris have to go through that? Dr. Brooks said that it is up to the oncologist (that's a doctor who specializes in cancer), but that the rule of thumb is that if more than 4 lymph nodes were involved, chemotherapy and radiation are usually recommended. This concurred with Dr. Loman's assessment.

Dr. Brooks wanted to know if Dr. Loman had done a full work-up, consisting of a bone scan (to see if cancer has spread to her bones), a CT-scan (to see if cancer had spread to her organs), and a specialized blood test.

We told her about the bone scan scheduled for the following Monday, and that the other tests had not yet been ordered.

Then we told her about Dr. Loman's comments on reconstruction, which wouldn't even begin for over a year, and which would involve two additional surgeries, weekly injections, and result in implants that would have to be replaced in 10 to 15 years. We asked her if this was the way these things were normally done.

Dr. Brooks told us that that was a pretty standard procedure for implants, but that there was another option. She said that not every institution offered it, but they had done it successfully at UCLA for several years.

The procedure is called a "TRAM-flap" reconstruction. (TRAM is an acronym for "Transverse Rectus Abdominus

Myocutaneous.") Simply put, it involves taking tissue from the abdomen and inserting it into the breast. The mastectomy and reconstruction are both done during the same surgery and involves four days in the hospital, whereas the mastectomy alone is considered an outpatient procedure.

We had gotten advice from several credible resources to be sure that whoever does any kind of surgery has done that procedure at least 50 times. Based on that advice Chris asked her, "How many times have you done this here? 50? 100?"

Dr. Brooks looked her right in the eye and said, matter-of-factly, "Thousands. We've done thousands of TRAM-flap reconstructions here."

Whoa! We were impressed.

"This seems like it's basically a cosmetic procedure. Will insurance cover it?" I asked. Sure, I'm willing to do just about anything for Chris, but I really didn't want to have to sell the house and cash in all of our retirement for this: two teams of surgeons, four days in the hospital, yikes!

Dr. Brooks asked who our insurance carrier was and, when we told her, said that there was a lot of paperwork but that Blue Cross was very good and would cover it.

Then we asked if it would be a problem that we lived so far away in the event that something unexpected happened following the surgery. She told us that people come to UCLA for medical care from all over the world, and go home afterwards. If there is a problem, their local doctors can work with UCLA doctors over the phone. As a matter of fact, we aren't really all that far away and could even come in if we needed to. After all, a two-hour drive isn't all that far compared to someone who would have to come in from, say, Connecticut!

Dr. Brooks then asked, "Would you like to talk to the plastic surgeon while you're here? I can see if he is available to see you right now."

Chris and I looked at each other. "Sure! Why not?"

Dr. Brooks disappeared for a few moments and Chris and I talked about this new development. She was kind of scared because it sounded like a lot to go through, but it also sounded like it would be a much better way to go in the long run. Basically, though, we were excited, relieved, and bewildered all at the same time. So many things to learn. So many things to verify with others.

Wonderful Dr. Brooks returned and said, amazingly, that Dr. Da Lio (pronounced "da-LEE-oh"), the plastic surgeon, could see us right now. It was the first of many times that we would see incredible teamwork and coordination at the Revlon/UCLA Breast Center.

We thanked her profusely and off we went to the fourth floor.

We waited, perhaps, five minutes and were shown into an examination room. A few minutes after that, in walked Dr. Da Lio. Like Dr. Brooks, he looked very young.

We talked for a few minutes and I was impressed that he already knew quite a bit about Chris's situation.

I told him, "Dr. Brooks said you've done this procedure thousands of times, but you don't look like you're old enough to have done *anything* thousands of times!"

He was a pretty reserved-type of guy, but he smiled. He explained the procedure to us just as Dr. Brooks had, telling us that he would take some tissue from her abdomen around her belly button giving her, in effect, a tummy-tuck (which she didn't need).

Chris said, in a mocking, pleading tone, "Can't you take it from my inner thighs instead??"

We all laughed and he said that they couldn't; she would have to be happy with the free tummy-tuck.

Chris was sitting in an examination chair, undressed from the waist up. Dr. Da Lio was sitting in front of her, gently pinching her abdomen from side to side and up and down around her belly button, testing the tissue to see if she was a good candidate for this procedure. He told us that she had "just barely enough" tissue for reconstruction of one breast.

Chris liked the "barely enough" characterization. "Bless your heart," she told him.

"If she gets hungry will her new breast gurgle?" I asked, trying to sound serious.

We all laughed again, and then Dr. Da Lio then told us about the risks. He said that chemotherapy wouldn't affect the reconstruction but that radiation might. He explained, "About 10 percent of these reconstructions can become distorted by radiation. If the distortion is severe, which is very rare in my experience, it cannot be fixed and you will have to live with it."

"So you mean," I asked him, "that considerably less than 10 percent would be distorted to the extent that we, as lay people, would notice it. Did I understand that correctly? In other words, some of that 10 percent would be distortions so minor that only you would see them."

He agreed.

"So the percentage of distortions that *we* would notice is even smaller than the 10 percent figure."

Right.

He said that you can only do this procedure once, and that if it got distorted it could not be fixed, even by an implant. We could do the TRAM-flap after radiation is finished in order to eliminate the possibility of distortion, but in the best of circumstances it would look like a patch because the skin would be discolored by radiation and the stretching and tissue replacement involved would make the new breast look different. He felt that, even with a little distortion, the end result would look better if she did it along with the mastectomy.

I realized immediately that there might also be a financial benefit to doing this procedure instead of implants. The TRAM-flap reconstruction is done at the same time as the mastectomy, therefore both procedures would be subject to the same deductible. If Chris decided to have the implants a year after the mastectomy, the implant procedures would occur in a different calendar year and would therefore be subject to a new deductible. Considering my deductible and maximum co-pay per year, that translated into about $4,000 that could be saved. The decision was entirely up to Chris because she was the one that had to endure the discomfort and live with the results, so I didn't even mention this to her. But the finances are still something for which I am responsible so I had to be aware of these things.

When we left Dr. Da Lio's office we had a lot to think and talk about. The big question was, of course, should we change ships and continue Chris's treatment at UCLA with wonderful Dr. Brooks and wonderful Dr. Da Lio? We were pretty excited about the possibilities, although we both felt some sort of allegiance to Dr. Loman even though we had a somewhat dark feeling about him. It's not that we didn't consider him competent, we just didn't feel as comfortable with his negative prognosis and the reconstruction options that he offered. Still, we felt like we might hurt his feelings if we chose to go to UCLA instead and, for some strange reason, we cared about that. In retrospect, that was a little silly of us, but that's the way we felt about it at the time.

It was clear that we needed some help making this decision, and we knew just the people we needed to ask: Anne and Ken.

Chris slept and I reflected during the long drive home. I had such a wonderful, peaceful feeling driving along and hearing Chris's deep breathing as she slept soundly in the back. I felt as though we were exactly where we needed to be, doing exactly what we needed to be doing, and that she was safe and warm, and that I was her protector.

May 19:
The Star Wars Incident

A ll of the recent events and their complications had caused my stress level to approach 'unbearable' and, as a result, my patience and tolerance for any kind of emotional stimulation was at an all-time low. This condition culminated in some surprising behavior on my part; surprising to Chris and even to myself!

Movies are one of the things that Chris and I have always enjoyed together. When we first started dating she used to keep track of the movies that we saw together; one year we actually saw over 100!

The Star Wars movies have always been among our favorites, although I have been much more excited about it than she. Our first date back in 1978 was to see the first one, although it was my 6th or 7th time to see it. I confess that, when Luke was flying through the trenches of the Death Star in order to shoot his proton torpedo and annihilate the empire, I used it as an excuse to hold her hand!

It was no small event for us, then, when Star Wars: Attack of the Clones was released on May 16. I could hardly wait to see it, but with all that was going on we just couldn't get away. Until Sunday (the 19th), that is, when we went to an afternoon screening at our local mountain movie theatre.

Frankly, I wasn't sure if I could handle the suspense that the movie would undoubtedly deliver, but I was hoping that I would become so absorbed that the stress of current events would slide to the background.

With high anticipation we sat in the theater just about dead center (for the best sound), munching on our popcorn waiting for the previews to begin. In the row in front of us next to the left-hand aisle sat four ladies who were talking and laughing with great enthusiasm.

I found it very annoying.

This was a movie theater, after all, and, as in a library, you just don't talk loudly. Ever. Even if there is nothing on the screen but a slide show of advertisements, you just don't do that. My wife had cancer. Our money situation was tenuous. I didn't have time to work much to try to fix that, and even when I did I just didn't feel like it. I was fighting depression. I didn't know what was going to happen. The movie was about to start; were they going to shut up so I could hear it? And so on...

As these women were carrying on, my tension was building to the breaking point. I tried to ignore them, but I just couldn't. I'm sure it was the stress, but I snapped and did something that I've never done before. It was almost a dream; as if I was just sitting there watching while someone else took over my body.

"EXCUSE ME," I yelled very sarcastically and very loudly, making much more noise, in fact, than the four of them put together. *"DO YOU THINK YOU COULD KEEP IT DOWN OVER THERE?"*

It was one of those moments where you could hear a pin drop as everyone in the theater froze. It might have been my imagination, but I think that even the popcorn at the concession stand stopped popping for a moment. I'm usually quite reserved and polite; I just don't do things like that. I could have walked over to them instead of yelling across the theater, but I didn't because I was overwhelmed to the point that I lost control.

Chris shrunk down in her seat with her hand over her face. "I know one of those women, Dave," she moaned. "She is in the Woman's Club with me. Thanks a lot." (It's unusual to go anywhere in our little community without seeing someone that we know.)

Yes, they quieted down. And yes, we enjoyed the movie a great deal. And no, the suspense didn't bother me. Star Wars, as usual, came through and did its job: we got lost in it and escaped our troubles for a couple of hours.

It just goes to show that the stress of dealing with cancer and all of its ramifications can lead you to some surprising behavior.

Pac-Man

It was about this time that we were introduced to the concept of "guided imagery." A combination of visualization and self-hypnosis, guided imagery is a mental technique where the patient forms an image in her mind that, in this case, will help the body fight cancer cells. Chris spent an hour with someone who specializes in this technique and came home with a new outlook and a new feeling of empowerment; there *was* something she could do to assist in her own treatment after all.

The idea was for her to form an image in her mind of familiar objects to represent the cancer cells and their destroyers. By associating these objects she could imagine the cancer cells' demise and, by doing so, use the proven but unidentified power of her own body. Chris is a very "right-brain" type of person and this was easy for her to do.

When she described this technique to me I immediately thought of the old Pac-Man video game of the 1980's, where the Pac-Man (who looked like a small yellow pie with a missing slice that represented a "mouth") moved around the game board under control of the player, gobbling up dots on the board as well as ghosts and other assorted objects. There were vivid sound effects that represented him chomping away and, since Chris and I often played that game early in our relationship, I knew that the music and sound effects would create a vivid image in her mind. If I could make an audiotape of those sounds, it would help her to imagine her body chomping up the cancer cells.

I remembered seeing a simulation of that game for the home computer, so I searched on the Internet and found a free version of the game that would run on my PC. I downloaded it and began to play, recording the sound effects as the game progressed. I played for about 20 minutes, then edited the recording to eliminate the quiet parts and the sounds of Pac-Man biting the dust to get about 10 minutes of positive-sounding Pac-Man effects. I then recorded it three times on a 30-minute cassette and she had a 30-minute tape of nothing but Pac-Man, eating up her cancer cells! She could listen to it in the car or when going to sleep, creating vivid images in her mind of the cancer cells being destroyed.

She also created her own imagery, with Emma (our baby standard poodle), Poncho (the parrot), and Lily (the cat that 'talks' like Arnold Schwarzenegger). Her vision went like this: Poncho and Lily sat on Emma's back while Emma ran around looking for cancer cells. When she found one, she stopped and Poncho and Lily jumped off and attacked. Poncho pecked at the cell and Lily urinated on it (after all, she is "The Urinator"), effecting its demise.

We'll never know if it really helped or not, but it served to give Chris a feeling of some control in an otherwise uncontrollable situation.

May 20:
The Bone Scan

We had to arrive for the bone scan at 10:00 a.m. That meant that we had to get the animals all taken care of and leave the house by 8:00. Kate, who normally doesn't work on Mondays, agreed to come in anyway to take care of everyone for us. When we arrived at Radiation for the scan, we were happy to see Georgia waiting for us in the lobby.

Today's festivities included a bone scan and a visit to Dr. Loman. The bone scan consisted of two steps. First, at the 10:00 appointment, Chris was injected with a radioactive dye. Then we had four hours to wait while the dye circulated in her system: the actual scan was at 2:00.

So, in order to pass the time, the three of us drove around a little and ended up at a Vietnamese restaurant where Georgia had had lunch while she was running her errands the day of the lumpectomy. This was quite a treat for us because we had never had Vietnamese food, and we enjoyed it very much.

We arrived back at the hospital by 2:00 for the scan, which took about 45 minutes. I had brought my computer so I could write some articles, but I didn't really get much done. I don't know why I lugged that darned thing around; I hardly ever used it, and when I did I got very little done because I normally only got small chunks of time, and by the time the computer warmed up I usually only had a few minutes before I was interrupted. I need more time than that to get focused enough on something to do anything worthwhile. Besides, I was usually too anxious or consumed with whatever was going on to concentrate.

Chris emerged from the scan and we all waited. We had been told that we would have to wait there for a while in case they wanted x-rays for clarification of something that they saw in the bone scan. Sure enough, a short time later a technician came in and told Chris that they wanted to take some x-rays. Our hearts sank; we naturally assumed that they saw something they didn't like, but Chris was brave, as usual, and got right up and followed him in there. After Chris was out of sight, Georgia started to cry and I just stared blankly at the floor. There was nothing to do but wait the few days for the results; it was a bit disconcerting.

We finally left the hospital at 3:30 and went to see Dr. Loman to find out what the tumor board had to say about Chris's situation.

Dr. Loman said that everyone was in agreement that a mastectomy was about the only option at this point, given the circumstances. He took a look at the drain, fiddled with it, and then, without warning, gently but firmly pulled it out! Chris looked at me with her mouth formed into a silent scream as if to say, *"OH, MY GOD!"* I could see why he hadn't prepared her for it because she probably would have tensed up and made it worse. I was amazed at how much tubing had been inside Chris... it had to have been at least 8 inches! She told me later that it hurt like hell, but only for a second, and then it was fine: sort of like ripping off a bandage, only worse.

Dr. Loman told us that he would begin the scheduling for the mastectomy and his scheduling nurse would be in touch.

The Big Decision

After we left Dr. Loman we went to see Ken at his office, which was only a couple of blocks away. Ken is such a good friend and wonderful all-around person; he was finished seeing patients for the day, and was doing paperwork and other things that busy doctors do, but he dropped everything, took the three of us into his conference room, shut the door, and said, "Tell me everything." And he *listened*. Even more importantly, just like Dr. Brooks, he *heard*.

We told him about the mastectomy and reconstruction options with Dr. Loman and at UCLA, and about our hesitation to move to UCLA because of Dr. Loman, and we asked him what sorts of things we should consider. The financial aspect was a non-issue because all parties involved accepted our insurance and our cost would therefore be the same no matter what we did. Besides, I wasn't going to impact Chris's treatment in any way, either real or imagined, because of the money. There were other issues, though, such as distance (in case of emergency), doctors, and the medical impact of the extra time involved in scheduling surgery.

Ken told us that there was a difference between "academic" medicine and "community" medicine. Academic medicine, in general, is on the leading edge and they try new things in order to make advances in the general science of medicine. There are pros and cons to this approach.

Community medicine is much more conservative in their treatments and technology and they don't adopt the latest methods until they have been thoroughly tested and proven by the academic folks. There are pros and cons to this approach as well.

> "... he knew how important it was for us to have confidence in our doctors and treatment plan."

He wanted to know how long these doctors had been in practice, where they were trained, and if they were "board certified."

"Don't they have to be board certified to practice medicine in California?" I asked him.

"No," he told me. "It's not the same as being licensed to practice, but a higher level of qualification."

While we were talking, Dr. Da Lio called on my cell phone, returning an earlier call from me. I had had a couple of questions about the TRAM-flap surgery and this was now an excellent opportunity for me to ask him the questions Ken had just raised: he was trained at UCLA, had been in practice at UCLA for seven years and yes, he was board certified.

Ken was very intense in his analysis of the situation, asking lots of questions about UCLA as well as our situation and how we felt about the whole thing. He finally said that he thought UCLA would be a better choice for several reasons, not the least of which was the fact that Chris had such a good feeling about them (Chris told Ken that every time that she entered the Revlon/UCLA Breast Center she felt like she was wrapped in a warm blanket of love and caring). Breast cancer is not Ken's field, but he does know medicine, patients, and related psychology and he knew how important it was for us to have confidence in our doctors and treatment plan. Besides, UCLA has long been considered one of the top medical institutions in the country and if we had the opportunity to take advantage of that resource, we should go for it. As far as Dr. Loman goes, Ken told us that doctors have to deal with physician changes all the time. It is not an affront and Dr. Loman would not take it that way. We have to do what's best for Chris; that was all that really mattered, and Dr. Loman would understand that.

We felt guilty, excited, and relieved all at the same time, but we still wanted to know more about Dr. Brooks based on Ken's questions.

The next day, I spoke to Mary Jo, Dr. Brooks' assistant, who told me that Dr. Brooks had been trained at Harvard where she stayed on as a Fellow for two more years, and she had been in practice for 8 years. When I asked if Dr. Brooks was board certified, Mary Jo said, "Oh, God yes!" I asked to have Dr. Brooks call us because I wanted to know if waiting a few weeks while arrangements were made at UCLA would make a medical difference for Chris.

Dr. Brooks called back that evening; just the sound of her voice on the phone was soothing to me. She said that another week or two would make no difference whatsoever.

It was time to decide. We both knew the right thing to do, so the next day I put another call in to Dr. Brooks who called back later that evening. I said, "Dr. Brooks, we have decided that we want you to do the mastectomy and Dr. Da Lio to do the TRAM-flap. Can you do that for us?" I was just a little intimidated because, for some reason, I felt that UCLA, being one of the best of the best, was somehow out of our reach, as we were just "mere mortals."

"I would be happy to do that for you," she told me. "I'll make all of the arrangements and when we have a date for surgery Mary Jo will contact you with the details."

She was so reassuring and I was so relieved that I began to get emotional. I barely choked out the words, "Thank you so much!"

"We'll take good care of her," she told me.

"I'm sure you will," I said, and meant it.

I'll never forget that two-minute conversation. I feel that it was a major moment in my life, mainly because of Dr. Brooks, her demeanor, and her genuineness. Maybe it was just that I needed so much to hear what she said to me, but

I can still hear her voice in the phone as clearly as I did that day.

We hung up and Chris and I hugged each other, literally jumping up and down; I couldn't maintain my composure. I felt like a huge weight had been lifted from my shoulders, not only because the decision had been made, but also because I knew it was the *right* decision. My Chris was going to get the best care available anywhere, from two doctors that we felt so very good about. I had learned that we had the freedom to change doctors if we felt it was in our own best interest.

Chris told me later that, at the time, she felt like she was boarding a scary ride at Disneyland. (She had said for some time that she felt that UCLA was the "Disneyland of Medical Centers" because she always felt so good when she was there.) She wasn't afraid, though, because she knew that at Disneyland they would never let anything bad happen to her, even on a scary ride.

The next day I was in sort of a quandary about when to call Dr. Loman's office to give them the news. We hadn't heard the results of the bone scan yet, and it seemed like it would be awkward to get those results after I told them that we were moving our care to UCLA. Call me silly, but I found the whole thing intimidating. Fortunately I didn't have to wait long.

That afternoon we got the call from Dr. Loman while I was in the shower. Dripping wet, I grabbed the phone and he told me that there were a couple of places that showed some degenerative disease ("arthritis") which is to be expected in a 49-year-old woman, but that there was no evidence that the cancer had spread into her bones. Great news!

The next day, I phoned Dr. Loman's office and spoke to

"I had learned that we had the freedom to change doctors if we felt it was in our own best interest."

---

his surgical coordinating nurse. I told her that we really appreciated everything Dr. Loman had done for us, but that we decided that we would be continuing Chris's care at UCLA. It was a very hard call for me to make because Dr. Loman had been the first doctor to treat Chris and had done an excellent job on the lumpectomy, but I was confident that it was the right thing.

His nurse couldn't have been nicer about it. "Thank you for letting me know," she said in a cheery voice. "Give Chris my best, and I hope that it all works out for you."

Done! We were going to UCLA!

June 3:
UCLA at Night

After our big decision had been made, the wait began for a surgery date. It took about a week for them to coordinate everything, which was no simple task. Getting even a tiny glimpse at what is involved in scheduling surgeries, I have a healthy respect for those who do it.

In our case there were three doctors involved: Dr. Brooks who would do the mastectomy, Dr. Da Lio who would do the TRAM-flap reconstruction, and an anesthesiologist. Then there was the operating room, recovery room, hospital room, and probably a lot of other things that we don't know about that had to be coordinated and scheduled.

It took about a week, but Mary Jo finally called with the date: June 13. Now we had to schedule all of the pre-operative testing and appointments. Since Dr. Brooks was in charge of the case, she ordered the remaining tests in the "workup" that she had asked about during our previous visit. Chris had already had the bone scan, but she also needed a special blood test and CT-scan so those were scheduled for June 3. Then appointments for both anesthesiology and Dr. Da Lio were made for June 10. Mary Jo was wonderful; realizing the distance that we had to travel, she scheduled things so as to minimize the number of trips that we had to make.

Then we discovered that UCLA offers a "multi-disciplinary" conference ("multi"). This process, which is mainly designed for patients who come there for a second opinion or who come from out-of-town, involves seeing doctors from different specialties, who then all sit down in the same room at the same time to discuss each case. There is a surgical oncologist (surgeon who specializes in cancer), medical oncologist (medical doctor who specializes in cancer), radiologist, psychologist, pathologist, etc. It sounded like the ideal thing for us, since we could get a good idea of everything that would be in store for Chris and, best of all, the different doctors would all discuss her situation in the same room. I instantly realized the value in this because each specialty views the facts of a case in light of their specific training. If any doctor disagreed with any of the others, they could iron out the differences immediately instead of through emails, voice messages, etc, which not only takes longer but is fraught with potential for errors and miscommunication.

We asked if we could participate and we were scheduled for June 12, the day before her big surgery. Perfect! They needed us to provide, in advance, all of the tissue specimens as well as the films from her bone scan, both of which were at the hospital where Dr. Loman had performed the lumpectomy. This did not present a big problem; I made arrangements to pick them up on the way to our next UCLA visit, which was June 3.

June 3 shaped up to be a complicated day. The only available appointment for the CT-scan had been for 8:00 p.m. (and would take two hours) but we had to drop off the bone scan films at the Revlon/UCLA Breast Center by 5:00 p.m. The lab was open until 6:00 p.m., and we had to drive through the worst possible traffic areas at the worst possible time of day. Complicating the situation was the fact that Chris wasn't supposed to eat anything for four hours before the CT-scan, which meant she was going to have to eat by 4:00 in order to avoid a sugar problem later.

Kate agreed to work late that day (until 5:00) so she could walk the dogs and feed everyone before she left. We left the house at 2:00 p.m. to pick up the bone scan films by 3:30, grabbed some tacos which Chris ate in the car before her 4:00 deadline, hit the rush-hour traffic (watching for those red lights in my rear-view mirror as we traveled the carpool lane with Chris asleep in the back) and, by the time we parked, walked (ran) into the building, and waited for the elevators, we arrived at the Breast Center at 4:59. Whew! It was a bit tense, but we made it.

The next stop was the lab for Chris's blood test; while she was in there, I wolfed down one of my tacos so she couldn't see; why make it more difficult for her when she can't eat? When we finished it was only 5:30, so we had 2 ½ hours to wait before the CT-scan. UCLA is only a couple of blocks from Westwood Village, a wonderful area of shops, movie theaters, and restaurants. Since we rarely get to this part of Los Angeles, we took a walk to enjoy the sights and sounds of the area.

As we approached one of the biggest theaters, it became obvious that something special was happening: it was the world premier of "The Divine Secrets of the Ya-Ya Sisterhood!" A great, big, old-fashioned Hollywood premier, complete with lights, TV cameras, celebrities, and limousines. What are the odds of *that*?? We stood there for a while and watched from across the street as Sandra Bullock, Ashley Judd, Susan Sarandan, and others arrived and walked the gauntlet of TV interviewers and photographers on their way into the theater.

We continued to walk around for a while, but the smell of all the different foods from restaurants of every description was too hard on Chris, who was getting pretty hungry. It was still only 7:00, so we decided to go back to UCLA and wait there. When we arrived, the technician was free because the patient who was scheduled just before Chris hadn't come.

That meant that he could take Chris immediately. Wonderful! First, he brought out a quart of some sort of goopy liquid that she had to drink in measured amounts every 10 minutes until it was gone. Chris expected the worst, but it was actually delicious, like a Pina Colada; cocoanut and pineapple. I wanted one too!

The test that Chris was having is commonly called a "CAT-scan" even though it is spelled "CT-scan", so when she finally went into the room for the scan I apologized to the technician and told him that we forgot to bring our cat. *I* thought it was funny, but I'm sure it was the first time he had heard it in at least an hour or so. He did, however, oblige me with a smile and courteous laugh.

He then put Chris on a table that moved through the center of a large machine with a big, round opening. It looked so big and she looked so small and vulnerable that my heart just wrenched. How can all of this be happening to my wife? I had to leave the room while they did the scan, and I left with tears running down my face. It was all just so *unfair.*

The test was over in about 15 minutes and we left about an hour earlier than we had expected, so we decided to go to our favorite delicatessen and have one of our favorite sandwiches. The deli was in Hollywood (about a 30-minute drive), right at the beginning of the famous Sunset Strip. What a treat! We hadn't been there in years, and the sandwich was wonderful. We split it and then split a piece of carrot cake; we rarely eat rich foods like that, especially that late, but comfort food was the order of the day and we felt that we had earned it.

It was another 90 minutes or so to get home. As usual, I enjoyed the serenity of the drive and the sound of Chris sleeping in the back. (It was late and there was no traffic, so I didn't use the carpool lane and therefore didn't have to worry about getting pulled over!) We got home about 12:15 a.m... it had been a long, complicated day, the first of several long, complicated days to come.

June 10:
The Pre-op, School, and Eclipse

The Saturday before the scheduled surgery, we made a dinner date with Gail and Sonia. We went to our favorite Mexican restaurant, but this time we were actually early! (I'm not quite sure how it happened, but it did.) We were seated at an oversized table and were positioned so that we were able to see the entrance to the restaurant.

As we munched on some chips and salsa, in walked a large stack of wrapped gifts, followed by another large stack of wrapped gifts. The two stacks were each so high that we could not see who was carrying them, but they were making their way toward our table. As they turned the corner to make their final approach, we could see the faces of Gail and Sonia behind their respective piles. One of them was even carrying a bag that contained more wrapped gifts in one of the hands that was supporting the boxes. We stopped chewing mid-chip and watched with amazement as they plopped the boxes down near Chris and joined us at the table.

"Are you kidding me?" said Chris in amazement. "What the heck is *this*??"

"We thought we'd get you a few things for your hospital stay," Gail told her.

"Once we got started, we couldn't stop," added Sonia. "We had so much fun!"

The generosity of these two women was simply amazing. Not only were they generous with their time, but with their hard-earned money as well. They had driven 80 miles (that's ea*ch way*) to a large shopping center and spent an entire day picking things out for her. I can't even imagine how much they must have spent, but one thing was for sure; it was not a trivial amount.

The loot included, among other things, three pair of pajamas (two of which were silk), a silk leopard-patterned robe, a couple of high-quality stuffed animals to keep her company (which, by the way, were ordered and shipped from a store in New York), several loose-fitting shirts to wear over bandages and dressings, and a nightgown. In total, there were 14 individual wrapped packages; I've never seen anything like it. We were both completely blown away, not only by the time and money they spent, but by the thoughtfulness of the gifts. It created quite a stir in the restaurant as all of these packages arrived coupled with our squeals of amazement and delight.

The following Monday, June 10, was going to be another long and complicated day. The multi-disciplinary conference was Wednesday with the big surgery the day after that. The day's agenda included lab tests, a pre-op (pre-operative) appointment with anesthesiology at 10:30, a pre-op appointment with the plastic surgeon at 11:30, a visit to Georgia's 4th grade class, and, since we were told Chris shouldn't have much to eat the night before surgery, an early last-blow-out-dinner-before-the-surgery meal at Lawry's The Prime Rib in Beverly Hills. I had to make arrangements for the animals because we would be gone so long, so Kate, once again, came in to work even though it wasn't one of her regular days, and came in late and stayed late so she could feed the dogs and horses before she went home. That way, the dogs would be alone for only a few hours between the time we left and the time she came in, and for only a few hours between the time she left and the time we returned home.

Georgia had told her students all about Chris's illness and had long wanted us to come for a visit. Since her school is in the general direction of UCLA we rarely got out there, so this was going to be an excellent opportunity to visit and meet the children. Besides, Georgia was going to retire in a few months so this would probably be our last opportunity as well. The children would go home at 2:30, our last appointment was at 11:30, and since it is only a 30-minute drive from

UCLA to the school I figured we could get there in plenty of time. Just to make sure, though, I wanted to get to UCLA early enough to do the blood work *before* the 10:30 anesthesiology appointment. Ha ha ha! We are famous for being late to *everything*, but everyone needs a dream, don't they??

Let's see... a two-hour drive in rush-hour traffic means at least 2 ½ hours to get there and we need to be there by 10:00 to do the lab work before the 10:30 appointment... we'll have to leave at 7:30. Ha ha ha! Hmmm... I have to shower, shave, check my email, walk the dogs, feed the horses, make breakfast... what the heck, I just won't go to bed at all!

Well, of course we left later than 7:30 and, between that and more traffic than I expected, we just barely got to UCLA in time for the lab work before the 10:30 appointment. *Barely.* (Chris slept on the way there, so if we had finally been pulled over in the carpool lane, we definitely would have been late!)

After the blood was taken, we rushed up to the pre-op appointment where Chris registered and I found a place in the waiting room. Just to be silly, I sat in a tiny little chair at a tiny little child's table. It wasn't very comfortable (the seat of the chair seemed to be about even with my ankles so when seated my knees were about even with my armpits) but I was going for the laugh so I hung in there until Chris found me. I got the laugh (well, it was smile at least).

It wasn't long until they called Chris so they could weigh her. When she got on the scale she closed her eyes, so the nurse asked her, "Don't you want to know how much you weigh?"

"No, I don't. I've been eating pie ever since I found out I had cancer!"

We finally ended up in an examination room with a nurse who was going to conduct the pre-op interview, at which time I discovered that Chris was supposed to have seen her regular doctor (Dr. Win) to get a surgical release. Since Dr. Win was over 2 hours away and the surgery was in three days with the multi-disciplinary conference the day before that, we only had one day to get the release completed, faxed, and approved. Ooops! Mr. "I'm-handling-all-the-details-so-Chris-doesn't-have-to" made a big boo-boo. The nurse was wonderful about it, though, and said that they could do the testing they needed right there, so out came the electrocardiogram (EKG) and they did the test right on the spot.

Then we went over Chris's medical history, previous surgeries, how she had reacted to previous anesthesia, etc. A lot of this was supposed to have been done at the doctor visit that I failed to schedule. I was surprised at how long it took, and we were rapidly approaching the 11:30 appointment. It soon became evident that we were going to be late, but the nurse that was talking to us knew about the other appointment, which I found to be very impressive. These people really had their act together! She called them to tell them we would be a little late and that took off some of the pressure, but we still had a boatload of stuff to do the rest of the day. And then we got the bad news: they hadn't done all of the required testing at the lab so we had to go back before we left. And, we needed to go to X-ray as well. Great; now we're going to be even later getting to Georgia's classroom.

Off we went to see Dr. Da Lio, the plastic surgeon, for our 11:30 appointment. When we got on the elevator, an orderly got on with us, pushing a laundry cart full of medical gowns, those loose garments that they ask the patients to put on ("opening to the front", or "opening to the back") so the doctor can waltz in and fling them off for the exam. Chris pointed into the basket and said, "I recognize that one; I wore it last week!" We all laughed.

We were about 15 minutes late but we only had to wait a few minutes. Very impressive; everyone knew about everyone else we were seeing and we didn't have to wait very long no matter where we went. It was obvious that there was a lot of coordination and teamwork behind the scenes.

Dr. Da Lio looked at Chris's stomach and took a marking pen to draw on her skin. He started at one hip and drew an

"I knew what a big difference I was making by handling the details."

upward crescent that went above her belly button and ended on her other hip, level with the beginning of the crescent. Then he did the same thing again but drew a downward crescent, again from hip to hip, starting and ending at the same points as the other mark he had just made. It looked sort of like a giant eye, with her belly button, in the middle of the two crescents, as the pupil! I told him that it was a very nice drawing, "but does it have anything to do with the surgery??"

He smiled, but didn't laugh; he struck me as the brilliant-and-serious type. He explained that the marks were where the incisions were going to be and I gasped quietly. I thought, "Good heavens! He's going to carve her up like a Thanksgiving turkey!" I don't think she understood the meaning of what he said, and, frankly, I was glad. Why worry her with the details? It was going to happen whether she knew about it now or not, so I wanted to spare her any worry that the details might cause; there I am, being protective again.

By now it was about 12:15 and we rushed down to the lab. On the way there, Chris asked me for the third time that day what we were doing and what was next; she was so focused on the cancer that she had trouble keeping the day's schedule straight. I found it somewhat amusing, but also gratifying because I knew what a big difference I was making by handling the details. In some ways I felt like a tour guide as she followed me around from appointment to appointment.

She took a number and had to wait for what seemed like an eternity. It really wasn't that long, but it felt like it because we knew that Georgia was expecting us and we were behind schedule. I called Georgia in her classroom to tell her we would be later than expected and she understood, but that didn't relieve any of my angst.

Next stop: X-ray. She put on a medical gown and then we waited in a small waiting area. We sat next to a very old man and his even-older friend. The younger of the two was friendly enough and asked Chris why she was there. When Chris told him, he said, "The problem with getting cancer as young as you are is that it spreads so quickly."

My gast had never been so flabbered. Talk about insensitive; what a thing to say to someone with cancer!! She laughed about it later and we wrote it off to semi-senility, but I think that down deep it bothered her just a little. I remember thinking, "No matter how much I do, I just can't protect her from everything."

I really dislike rushing around, but we were under the gun at this point. Not only did we have to get to Georgia's school before the children left, but we also had to make sure that Chris ate something before we got there. If she had another sugar problem it would have scared the you-know-what out of a room full of fourth-graders!

We hurried back to the car and headed for tacos and then the school. We arrived about 2:15 and only had a few minutes with the children before they went home. They had been studying China and, at Georgia's request, I had prepared a video from one of my eclipse trips showing some of the sights in and around Beijing. Some of the children really wanted to see the video, so they stayed after class and we all sat on the floor watching and talking about it. They were really sweet kids and we all had a good time. It was good to see Chris so relaxed and enjoying herself.

The school happens to be directly under the landing pattern for Los Angeles International Airport, so every few minutes a jet would fly about 100 feet overhead as it made its landing approach. Each time that happened, the entire building shook for a few seconds, although it wasn't very loud because it was well insulated, probably for that very reason. No one seemed to notice.

After the kids went home, the three of us hung around for a few minutes as Georgia straightened up her classroom. She took us on a short tour of the school… everything sure is smaller that I remembered from my own elementary school! I guess they changed the way they build them. Or maybe it's because I'm bigger now; yeah, that's probably it. (!)

It was about a 45-minute drive on surface streets to Lawry's, a restaurant that we just love but rarely go to. It is a two-hour drive from the mountains; we have been known to make the drive there just for dinner, then return home! But we hadn't done it in a long time so this was a big treat. We got there at 4:45, about 15 minutes before they started seating so we waited and had some appetizers. At 5:00 they seated us. (I had made reservations a week or so in advance; there's that try-to-think-of-everything-and-plan-ahead thing again.)

But wait! There's more!

It just so happened that there was going to be a partial eclipse of the sun that evening. This occurs when the moon moves in front of the sun but doesn't completely cover it. (A "total" eclipse occurs when the moon moves in front of the sun and *does* completely cover it.) During a partial eclipse, you must use eye protection at all times in order to observe it because the sun, even though some of it is covered, is much too bright to look at safely with the naked eye.

I am an absolute maniac when it comes to eclipses of the sun: as of that date, June 10, 2002, I had been to eight total solar eclipses and intended to go to every eclipse for the rest of my life no matter where they occurred. They are simply the most incredible thing that I've ever seen, and bring me a sense of peace, serenity, and awe that have no equal. It is such a moving and amazing experience that I am always re-

---

"I remember thinking, 'No matter how much I do, I just can't protect her from everything.'"

---

duced to sobbing uncontrollably whenever I see one.

My eclipse travels have taken me to Kenya, Hawaii, Paraguay, India, Mongolia, Aruba, Romania, and Zambia. Chris has been to two eclipses with me: Hawaii and Aruba. She found the eclipse experience to be wonderful, but she is not as enthusiastic as I am so she only goes to eclipses that are in places that she wants to visit. If she doesn't want to go to wherever an eclipse will be happening, she is happy to take me to the airport and take care of the animals while I'm gone; she says that I have made her dreams come true and she certainly wants mine to come true as well, so she would never stand in the way of one of my eclipse expeditions. Fair enough.

As you can tell, I am serious about this!

Normally my fanaticism for eclipses is limited to total eclipses. Partial eclipses are interesting, but not as thrilling as total eclipses. (I have traveled halfway around the world to see a total eclipse, but wouldn't travel very far to see a partial.) When it's in my own backyard, though, of course I'm going to check it out, so I had brought several pair of the special glasses required to view it. It would first be visible at about 5:15, so at 5:16 I went outside and looked. Sure enough, there was a small bite taken out of the sun's disk! I was thrilled and went back bubbling over with excitement.

Georgia had never experienced an eclipse, so she and Chris took the glasses and went outside to look. They, too, were excited to see it. We ordered our meals and had a great time, except that every 10 minutes or so one of us had to go outside to check the progress of the eclipse. I went, sometimes Georgia went, and sometimes Chris. Between the three of us leaving to check the eclipse, our table seemed in constant motion.

Our server asked us what we were doing and when we told her, she wanted to borrow the glasses and take a look as well. She did, and returned with a busboy who also wanted to borrow the glasses, and he said that the cooks wanted to borrow them too! Before long, the manager came over and wanted to borrow them, and the atmosphere in the restaurant became pretty festive as everyone got excited about the eclipse.

Then some of the other people who were dining in the restaurant became aware of the eclipse and the special glasses, and they wanted to borrow them to go have a look! Chris even got up and went over to a large party and told them about it and offered the glasses; most of them took her up on it. People from all over the restaurant were parading outside to see this eclipse and it made my heart sing to see so many people enjoying the wonders of our solar system.

In addition to the eclipse excitement, we were celebrating Father's Day. Even though we have no human children, Chris and I always honor each other on Mother's Day and Father's Day because of the roles we play with our many animals. Seeing as how Chris would be in the hospital on Father's Day, which was the following weekend, she wanted to give me my gifts that evening. In spite of all that Chris was going through and the fact that she was going to have major surgery in a couple of days, she still had it together to wrap a few gifts and a couple of cards and bring them to the restaurant. I was very touched.

When the bill came, we were told that dessert was on the house because we were so nice to let them use the glasses!

The ride home was just as wonderful as it always was; sleep for Chris, serenity for me, light traffic, and no carpool lane. Another long, complicated, *and very successful* day was over.

June 12:
The Multi-Disciplinary
Conference

The most dangerous part of our journey was about to begin. This was the basic plan: today, Wednesday, we would attend the multi-disciplinary conference. We would spend the night near the hospital at Gail's city home and then Thursday morning report to the hospital at 5:30 a.m. (!) for Chris's mastectomy and TRAM-flap reconstruction surgery. She would be in the hospital for four days, and probably be released the following Monday depending, of course, on how quickly she recovered. Since Chris was in excellent health (besides the cancer, that is), we all expected the surgery to go about as well as it could. Of course that was easy for me to say; I wasn't the one going under the knife!

There was already a fly in the ointment, however. The evening before we were to leave I got a call from the anesthesiology coordinator who told me that they didn't like the way Chris's electrocardiogram looked and they would not do the anesthesia without approval from a heart specialist.

"We can't possibly see a heart specialist because we are 2 hours away and will be at the multi all day tomorrow," I told her with a sinking feeling. The stress of the situation made me feel like my insides were shrinking inside my skin. The possibility of not doing the surgery was one thing, but what about her heart? Was there something wrong with it? How are we going to juggle all of this? It was one of the most stressful moments of this entire ordeal.

The coordinator told me that she would see what she could do, but that it was too late to arrange anything that day.

She would do it first thing in the morning and call me. My hopes were not high, because I know how complicated scheduling can be. UCLA is a large organization and I just didn't think that any institution of that size would be "limber" enough to be able to coordinate everything that needed to be done. But then again, there was nothing I could do about it, so I tried to just relax and wait until morning. I gave the co-ordinator our cell phone number and just hoped that we'd have a good signal when she actually called.

The multi was supposed to begin at 9:00 which meant, with traffic, etc. we would have to leave the house at, gulp, 6:30. Ha ha ha!

Again, it was wonderful Kate to the rescue. Not only did she move into the house for the five days we would be at UCLA, but she did most of my morning chores so I didn't have to do them before we left. We left pretty much on time, and had a pretty uneventful ride into town during the morning rush hour.

We were about 15 minutes from UCLA when the anesthesiology coordinator called on the cell phone. She had gotten Chris an appointment at 1:00 with a cardiologist whose office was in the building next to the building where the multi would be, and the folks at the multi were notified that we would be leaving and then returning. They said it wouldn't be a problem; what an incredible place UCLA was.

I wanted to hug her over the phone. My skepticism was creeping in, though, and I wondered if it would really go as smoothly as I hoped. There were a lot of people in many different offices and departments that had to have their act together in order for this to work. We would see.

When we got to the Revlon/UCLA Breast Center, where the multi was held, there was Georgia waiting for us. What a good sister! She really had come through during all of this and rearranged her life many times so she could be there to support Chris, and me as well. It meant a lot to me, and I know that it also meant a lot to Chris.

There were six other patients involved in the conference. We all gathered in the main conference room to discuss what would be happening during the day, which would play out like this: each patient would be assigned an examination room and the doctors from the various disciplines would rotate from room to room so that every patient would be able to talk to every doctor. Then, we could all go to lunch while the doctors assembled in the conference room and discussed each case in a forum-like setting. When they were through, one doctor would go to each room and discuss the findings and conclusions. It sounded like a pretty straightforward and intelligent approach.

Our examination room, with soft lighting and wood paneling, had a tape recorder and a blank cassette so we could record whatever we wanted to. I didn't need to use it, though, because I had brought my own as usual, but I had to admire UCLA's thoroughness and thoughtfulness.

The doctors started coming in and it soon became apparent just how organized and 'together' they really were, because each one commented on the fact that 1) Chris's surgery was going to be the next day and 2), that we had to leave for a 1:00 appointment for cardiac testing. I was relieved and amazed that this complication was really going to go well after all.

At one point, a psychiatrist came in to see Chris to, presumably, evaluate her mental condition and offer assistance if she was having a problem with fear and/or anxiety. After talking with us for about five minutes, I got the distinct impression that he was a bit perplexed at our attitudes in general, and Chris's attitude in particular. We were laughing and joking and ended up talking to him about Dr. Da Lio; it turned out that the psychiatrist had had Dr. Da Lio perform a small procedure to remove a scar on his forehead, and he proudly showed us the results, which were impressive. He bore a striking resemblance to Henry Winkler, the actor who played

"The Fonz" on Happy Days, so we felt like we were talking to The Fonz instead of a doctor!

At about 15 minutes before 1:00 an assistant to Dr. Brooks came in and told us that we had better leave in order to get to the cardiac appointment on time. Amazing.

When we arrived at the cardiologist's office, they were expecting us. We did have to wait a bit because they had sort of "squeezed us in" to their schedule, but when we finally saw him he not only had all of Chris's records, but he was aware that we were in the middle of the multi and needed to get back! I was *very* impressed.

The cardiologist did an exam and several tests, one of which (the "echocardiogram") showed a picture of Chris's heart beating on a video screen. Chris also had to do a treadmill test, where they hook about 11 electrodes up to various places and then have her walk at various speeds on a treadmill to get her heart pumping. Because she was in such excellent physical condition, she was conversing and joking with them throughout the entire test. (Chris gets more exercise than that every day tending to the horses and chores around our property, and at an elevation of 5,800 feet! This test was easy for her.) We later found out that some people have had to stop the test because they get too winded. The doctor and technicians just sort of rolled their eyes and said, in effect, "There's certainly no problem here!" She got her surgical clearance and the doctor told her, "Good luck. You are wonderful; everything is going to be just fine."

By the time we got back to the multi the doctors were finished with their conference and were going back into the various exam rooms to deliver the results. There was a knock on the door and in walked Dr. Linnea (pronounced li-NAY-a) Chap, the oncologist that we had requested. Gail and Sonia had heard good things about her and, as it turns out, my accountant's wife had finished breast cancer treatment the previous year and Dr. Chap had been her oncologist. Everyone raved about her so we had requested her specifically; we were not disappointed. Just as with Dr. Brooks and Dr. Da Lio, we liked her as soon as she walked in the door looking youthful, slender, full of confidence, and with a big smile on her face. It was our first conversation with an oncologist, so we would finally get to find out what the total treatment package would entail, and the timing as well.

The first thing that she told us was that the consensus of the group was that the next day's procedure was exactly what Chris should be having. All of the tests had been re-evaluated (there's that second opinion again… or was it the third??) and based on those results there was really very little discussion. Everyone agreed.

That was great news, and Georgia, Chris and I all felt good about what was going to happen. Dr. Chap then laid out her preliminary view of a treatment plan.

Dr. Chap would be recommending both chemotherapy and radiation. She explained that chemotherapy is considered "systemic," meaning that it treats her entire body whereas radiation is considered "local," meaning that it treats one specific area of the body. The chemo was going to be necessary because six out of the 14 lymph nodes that had been removed tested positive for cancer. This indicated that cancer cells had been introduced into the lymph system that, theoretically, could have transported them to other parts of her body. The tests (bone scan, CT-scan, and blood work) showed no indication that this had happened, but there was still a good possibility that some bad cells were floating around and chemotherapy was intended to knock them out.

The chemo would begin about a month after the surgery, and would be once every three weeks for six treatments. (Yes, her hair would fall out, but it *would* grow back.) Then, four to six weeks following the last chemo treatment Chris would begin radiation therapy, which would consist of one treatment every day, Monday through Friday, for six weeks.

Yikes!

"... so I told myself, 'There's nothing you can do about that one, so don't go there 'til you get there'."

It wasn't happy news, but it was important news because now we could at least get an idea of what life would be like in the foreseeable future and could plan accordingly. It's a funny thing about bad news: even if it's worse than you thought it would be, knowing is better than not knowing because at least you know what you're up against. It's that "information is power" thing again: uncertainty makes any bad situation worse, so the more information you can get and the sooner you can get it, the better off you will be.

My mind immediately started working on the treatment schedule that lay ahead. Six chemotherapy treatments three weeks apart meant 15 weeks between the first and last one. If that started around the middle of July, it should be over around the end of October. That meant that radiation would begin around the beginning of December, continuing roughly through the middle of January. Whew!

As my mind raced through the possible scenarios, there were suddenly several concerns. First of all, how were we going to go to UCLA every day for six weeks for radiation? Two hours each way, plus traffic and treatment; we're talking about a full-time job here! Not to mention the expense of gas, wear and tear on the car, parking, lunch, etc. Maybe Chris could stay at Georgia's house every other night and drive one way each day. She wouldn't want to be away from her animals that much, so that wasn't an option. I quickly came to the conclusion that we'll probably have to get the radiation somewhere closer to home, providing that there was no compromise in the quality of care. But where? There was some research in my immediate future.

One thing was sure; no matter where we ended up for radiation, it would involve driving down the mountain every day. December and January are potential weather months in the mountains, including fog, falling and fallen rocks, snow, wind, and rain. Driving is always treacherous. How was Chris going to get down the mountain? As I thought about that one, I could feel the stress shrinking my body inside my skin again, so I told myself, "There's nothing you can do about that one, so don't go there 'til you get there."

I snapped back to the conversation at hand and Dr. Chap was talking about a research program they were conducting and we were invited to participate. We said we'd consider it, so the coordinator for the project came in and proceeded to go over the details, reading from a document explaining everything in great detail. The document was about 50 pages, and it took almost 2 hours!! By the time she was finished our heads were spinning, and we left for dinner.

Originally we had been told that Chris shouldn't eat anything but clear broth the night before the surgery, but Kathleen, Dr. Da Lio's nurse, had come for a short visit during the multi and she told us that it would be all right to eat rice, chicken, etc. as long as it wasn't a really heavy meal. Hooray! Japanese, here we come!

We had a great meal at a local sushi bar, and Chris was able to enjoy some Miso soup, several pieces of sushi, and a chicken and rice dish. It was just perfect for her and for us as well. Considering what she was going to be going through the next day, Chris was perfectly calm and normal; I think I would have been a basket case had I been in her position.

After dinner, Georgia went home and we went to Gail's, getting to bed early because we had to be at the hospital by 5:30 a.m., which meant we had to get up around 4:30.

Another long, very complicated, but successful day.

June 13:
Mastectomy and Reconstruction

Getting up at 4:30 wasn't so bad; it sure is quiet at that time of day! Chris didn't really have that much to do to get ready since she was not supposed to wear any makeup and there was no point in getting dressed. She selected a pair of her new silk pajamas and her new robe to wear to the hospital and we were ready to go right on time. Just before she put them on, however, she looked down at her right breast, knowing that she would never see it quite that way again.

"You've been a good boob all these years," she said. "I'm sorry this is happening to you, but it's not your fault."

I wasn't sure if she was joking or not, but it was sweet.

We actually arrived at the hospital on time, parked in the underground lot and made the long walk to the lobby. About halfway there, Chris stopped suddenly and said, "Oh, no!"

I was startled. "What??"

"I forgot to bring my boob!"

I laughed out loud. How could she be in such a good mood? I was apparently more nervous than she was!

I said, "What do you mean? *I'm right here!*"

We walked into the lobby at about 5:35 and there, bless her heart, was Georgia, reading a book. She looked up with sleepy eyes and told us that she had been there for 30 minutes: the traffic had been much lighter than she expected.

It was about 45 minutes until they called us to do the paperwork and make the financial arrangements. We got into the pre-op area about 7:00. Chris was in the required gown and on her gurney in just a minute or so and then the wait began for her 7:30 departure for the operating room.

I asked her if she felt nervous and she said she didn't. Yet. About 7:10, much to our surprise, Sonia appeared. She had been so worried about her "Chrissy" that she left her house in the mountains at 4:00 in the morning, hit quite a bit of traffic, and, much to her relief, found her way to Chris's bedside in time to see her before she went in. We were all blown away by that extreme effort and I was struck with the warm feeling of support that *I* felt. It is important to support the patient, but the partner/caregiver also needs support and I hadn't been consciously aware of that until that moment. Sonia is truly a treasure; I'm sure that Gail would have been there as well had she not had patients to see that morning.

A few minutes later, Dr. Brooks popped in to say hello, and to make sure that everything was okay. We had been hoping she would because we really liked her and any excuse for a visit was okay with us! She explained that there would be two teams working on her at the same time. Dr. Brooks and her team would be doing the mastectomy while Dr. Da Lio and his team were "harvesting" the tissue from her abdomen. (I thought that term was a little graphic, considering the situation!) When Dr. Brooks was finished, she would leave and Dr. Da Lio would be inserting the harvested tissue into her breast while the rest of his team closed up her abdomen. What a process! I'm not sure if I felt better or worse knowing all of that, but I was glad that I had a picture in my mind.

Dr. Brooks' portion of the procedure would take about an hour but the entire procedure would take about six hours, and then Chris would be in recovery about an hour before we could see her. Dr. Brooks told us where to wait so that she could find us when she was finished.

We took some photos to remember the moment, Dr. Brooks left to get ready, and then the nurse arrived to insert an IV in preparation for the anesthesia.

A few minutes later a woman arrived and introduced herself as Chris's anesthesiologist. She asked some questions about how much Chris had in her stomach, etc. and then injected something into the IV to "help Chris relax." I knew that Chris would soon be fading away into la-la land, and Chris knew it too. I asked her if she was nervous and she said she was. We looked at each other and, as before her previous surgery, I told her I loved her, that I would be as close as I could be every second, and that I'd be at her side as soon as they let me. I tried to hide my tears but I don't think I did a very good job. We kissed and I stroked her forehead and noticed her eyes were starting to glaze over a bit and her speech was getting slurred. She was 'gone'.

It wasn't long before they came and wheeled her away. Georgia, Sonia, and I walked along side her as long as we could, but when that last door closed behind her I completely broke down. I wasn't really worried that something bad would happen, it was just so horrible that she had to go through all of this, she seemed so vulnerable, and it was just so damned unfair. I leaned against the wall and sobbed uncontrollably; I was completely unaware of Sonia or Georgia or how they were handling it.

I finally collected myself and the three of us went back to the lobby and waiting area. We decided to go for a walk and have some breakfast, so the three of us walked into Westwood Village, past the theater where Chris and I had seen the movie premier, to a local deli. Time to pile on the comfort food, and believe me, I didn't hold back. There were no health considerations whatsoever; I ate everything and anything that helped me to feel better. It wasn't pretty. It was tasty, but it wasn't pretty!

After breakfast, feeling a little more relaxed we returned to the waiting area to wait for Dr. Brooks to arrive following the mastectomy portion of the surgery. About an hour and a half after the surgery began, she found us and said that everything had gone extremely well and she was optimistic that they had been able to get all of the tumor.

Now the serious waiting began. Dr. Da Lio's nurse, Kathleen, had taken my cell number and promised to call with progress reports, which she did. Her calls were comforting and I was grateful that she was so caring to take the time.

"Everything is going well. Now they are closing the harvest area."

"Everything is fine. Dr. Da Lio is working under the microscope now."

"We will be finished in about 30 minutes. You will be able to see her in about an hour and a half."

In the meantime, Georgia had to leave for an appointment and told us she would be back in a couple of hours, so Sonia and I stayed in the waiting area just talking and passing the time. At one point, we both went to our cars in the parking garage and took a nap; I had been up since 4:30, and she had been up since about 2:00, so we were both pretty tired. We connected again about an hour later and went to the hospital cafeteria for lunch.

During lunch, Sonia and I talked about lots of things but I found myself thinking about getting Chris home after she was released. How would she be able to get into the 4Runner with an incision from hip-to-hip? How would she handle over two hours in the car? Come to think of it, it would be in the middle of the day, so there would probably be a lot of traffic. And so on...

Then I remembered my own wise words: "Don't go there 'til you get there." There was nothing I could do at that moment that would affect that scenario; whatever was going to happen would happen, so there was no point in wasting even an ounce of energy on it. Easy to say, but hard to do.

When we returned to the waiting room, we sat near a woman who was sleeping on a couple of the chairs. She looked familiar but I didn't really put it together until she woke up and we started talking: she was an actress that I'd seen in many films, including The Witches of Eastwick. She couldn't have been any nicer, and we had a nice time talking with her about some of the films she had worked on and about her husband, for whom she was waiting while he underwent surgery.

I was getting a little impatient waiting for the call that told us we could see Chris, so when I went to the desk for the umpteenth time to ask, the woman told me that she was probably on the fifth floor and we should just go up there. So we did.

When I walked into the room, my heart sank and rose at the same time. Her chest was all wrapped up, she was wearing an oxygen tube, her mouth was open and her eyes were closed, there were machines hooked up to her that were beeping and blinking, her hair was a mess, her lips were dry and cracked, and her face was white as a sheet.

As I approached the bed, she half-opened her eyes and looked at me with a bleary half-aware expression, managing a weak smile. I gently stroked her forehead and said, "You are the most beautiful thing I've ever seen." I wasn't sure if she could understand the words because I was having a tough time choking back tears, or if she would even remember them considering the fact that she was still coming out of the anesthesia. I thought that she probably wouldn't be feeling her most attractive, and I wanted her to know that I thought she looked wonderful. (As it turns out, she *did* hear me and remembered it too.)

She indicated through hand gestures and some weak whispers that her mouth was very dry and she was too hot, so I went to the nursing station and they showed me where the ice machine was, along with cups and "sponges-on-a-stick", which were little lime-green sponges about the size of a dime at the end of a stick about 4 inches long. I hurried back to her side and used the sponges to wet her lips and tongue. She was not supposed to drink any water but this extremely small amount was acceptable, so that was my job for the time being. Every now and then I fed her a few chips of ice with a spoon (the nurses told me that was also okay).

The first day or so it was not uncommon for her to ask for the ice chips and then fall asleep before I was able to put them in her mouth. Or, when I did put them in her mouth she would doze off before they could melt and she could swallow them. I had to wake her up so she wouldn't choke; I felt fairly confident that coughing would not be a good thing for her to be doing at that stage in her recovery.

Bedridden patients have a tendency to get blood clots in their legs because they cannot walk around. The solution to this problem is a device that consists of compression sleeves placed on each leg, which are attached to an automatic pump. The sleeves are similar in principle to the cuffs used to take blood pressure. At timed intervals, the pump is automatically activated and slowly fills the sleeves with air, causing the legs to be compressed after which the air is released, relieving the compression. This periodic squeeze-release, squeeze-release process results in better blood circulation through the legs.

Chris was wearing these devices on her legs, and every 15 minutes or so the pump would come on for a few minutes, followed by a gentle "whoosh" as the air was released. I found that sound to be reassuring, as it was yet another machine that was taking care of her.

It wasn't too long before Georgia returned, having found us after a little detective work. She and I then took turns with the sponge and ice chips, and Chris just "existed" in the bed.

Every hour for the first 24 hours the nurses had to check Chris's reconstructed breast to make sure that the blood was flowing properly through the veins that the surgeon had connected, under the microscope, to the transplanted tissue. They did this by placing a microphone-like device against the skin and moving it around until they could hear "PSHEW, PSHEW, PSHEW" which was the sound of the blood as it was pumped through the veins. As long as it sounded like that, everything was in good shape.

This surgery left her with four (count 'em "F O U R") drains; one each coming out of the side and bottom of her breast and two just below her new belly button. (I guess we had better brush up on our lyrics to "Oh! Canada!") This wasn't a surprise because it was in the pre-operative information that they had given us (it had been a surprise *then*!) but it was surreal to see them all pinned to her bedding. Naturally the nurses checked the output from the drains and emptied them, but they didn't sing when they did it (!) although I don't think that Chris was in any shape to care. Come to think of it, I don't think she was even aware of them doing it for the first two days or so.

They also checked her urine output. Since she was unable to get out of bed, it was necessary for her to have a catheter and the urine was collected in a bag that hung from the bottom of the far side of the bed. The amount of urine that was collecting in the bag was important for medical reasons, so they kept an eye on it; the more the better. Chris later observed, "You know your life has taken an unusual turn when you are excited that your urine bag is filling up."

The two biggest problems Chris faced in that bed were thirst and heat. It was important to keep her warm to keep the blood flowing those first critical hours, but she wasn't used to much heat, especially considering the fact that we were accustomed to a cooler climate in the mountains. We both have a pretty low heat tolerance, so I sympathized with her. It was only the areas around the incisions that had to be kept warm, so if we fanned her face that would be okay.

Chris had purchased a number of battery-operated mini-fans to keep the dogs cool when they were in the car. Three of the min-fans just happened to be in the car, so I went to get them and we put them on her tray table pointing at her face. When all of them were going, it helped her quite a bit and, although it made her thirst worse, she felt much more comfortable. I also retrieved "Haw," a beautiful stuffed Saint Bernard that our sweet friends Melissa and Jerry had given Chris to keep her company in the hospital.

About an hour after we were reunited with Chris, I felt a cold begin. It's funny how that works, at least with me. There is usually one specific point in time when I get that first spark of discomfort, usually a sore throat. And "Ping," there it was, and I knew I was getting sick. That's just great. Not only am I going to feel miserable during this crucial time in my life, I have to be doubly careful not to get Chris sick. A cold is bad news when you live in the mountains because the congestion can prevent your ears from adjusting to the change in altitude when you drive down to the city. Going *up* the mountain, however, is not a problem so I mentally figured out that by the time I had to drive down again the cold would be better. *That* was a good thing at least.

Sonia finally left about 6:00, looking pretty tired. What a sweet lady she was to have driven all that way in the middle of the night; friends like that are priceless. I remember thinking, "We certainly have some good ones, don't we?"

Georgia left shortly after Sonia did, but I was bound and determined to stay at Chris's side all night. She was fading in and out of sleep, so there wasn't a whole lot for me to do. I had brought my computer to try and do some work, but it just sat there; I barely had enough energy to go to the bathroom much less do any work. Besides, I had to keep getting up for sponge and ice duty.

Chris's room was large enough for four beds, two on the left and two on the right as you walked in. There was only one bed on each side; Chris's was on the right. The other space on her side was empty, which gave us lots of room but no place to sleep! (There was also only one bed on the other side of the room, occupied by a woman who had just had a *double* mastectomy with reconstruction.

There was a waiting room down the hall, which had a number of seats against the walls. The seats were configured so that there was an armrest for every two places, which meant that I couldn't comfortably stretch out. Around midnight I tried to get comfortable in there and was just falling off to sleep when a security guard came in to check on me. He was very nice, but wanted to know who I was and why I was there. It was good to know that the hospital had good security and that Chris was protected.

I just couldn't get comfortable or sleep more than 20 minutes at a time, so I gave up and went back in to see Chris. She was awake and encouraged me to go back to Gail's and get some sleep in a real bed; she would be fine and didn't want to have to worry about me.

I looked at the clock: it was about 1:30 a.m. and I knew I had to go or I would be worthless the next day. I left her bedside with great reluctance, and even though it was late and I was tired and Gail's house was only 10 minutes away, I was so anxious and full of guilt for leaving her that I didn't get to sleep until almost 3:00 a.m.

The next morning, by the time I woke up, showered, and stopped for breakfast, I didn't get to the hospital until 11:00 a.m. As I walked into the room I heard "PSHEW, PSHEW, PSHEW," that wonderful sound of blood flowing freely through the reconstruction as the nurse was positioning the little microphone "just so." Chris looked much better, greeting me with a smile, albeit a sleepy one. I was very relieved to hear that sound and to see that smile.

It turned out, though, that I had missed the big event of the day. A physical therapist had arrived and had gotten Chris to sit up on the edge of the bed; she had even walked a few steps! That effort had completely exhausted her and she had been asleep, even though they were checking her blood flow.

I spent the day getting ice chips, moistening her lips with the sponge, and keeping the fans running to keep her face cool. She still had to keep the area of the surgery warm with blankets to help the blood flow to the area, so the fans on her face were critical to her comfort. It soon became apparent that I was going to have to buy more batteries for the fans, so I planned a trip to the store. There were some things she wanted from the car and I needed to have lunch, so it was all coordinated so I could make the most of my time away from her. She had been given clearance to have some clear broth and Jello, so I helped her with that when it arrived, and it tasted soooooo good to her.

She continued to doze on and off and that was just fine with me; I enjoyed seeing the peaceful look on her face when she was sleeping, and hearing the sounds of the machines that were monitoring her. Besides, my cold was settling in and I needed the rest myself. It was pretty quiet in the room, except for the occasional sound of the leg compression pump and the sound of her breathing.

At one point I noticed a long pause between Chris's breaths as she was sleeping. The pause seemed to be a little too long and was making me uncomfortable, so I went out into the hall to find someone to check it out for me. I figured that it was better to ask and be wrong, than to *not* ask and be wrong. As luck would have it, one of the plastic surgeon interns was walking by and I asked him about it. He came in and told me that I was correct and that it indicated she was getting a little too much morphine, so he adjusted her dosage and her breathing became more regular. He told me that he was impressed with my observation.

"Good work," he told me. "Most people wouldn't have noticed that. Don't ever hesitate for even a second to ask someone if you see anything that doesn't seem right to you."

It felt good to hear that I had that kind of support, and to know that I had done something really important in the care of my wife.

Georgia arrived about 3:30, as soon as she could after her students went home. It was great to see her and to get some help with my fan, sponge, and ice chip responsibilities. A short time later, Hans and Joan arrived for a surprise visit. Hans and Joan are good friends of ours from the mountains who also have a home in the city. They were going to San Diego that day and the hospital wasn't far out of their way so they stopped by; we hadn't seen them in a long time so it was good to catch up a bit, although Chris wasn't in the best shape to receive visitors.

By 11:00 that night I was pretty tired and Chris was sleeping most of the time anyway, so I waved goodbye (didn't want to get too close with my cold and all) and left. I decided that I needed to be proactive about my cold and I remembered something that I used to eat as a bachelor when I got sick: steak and broccoli. When I wasn't feeling well I had steak and broccoli and then went right to bed so the food could work its magic. It seemed to work very well for me, and I had used this technique in Egypt two days before an eclipse when I got sick and was afraid that it would affect my experience. The next day I had been much better.

I found a little all-night coffee shop and told the server what I wanted, and a few minutes later a plate appeared on which was a perfectly cooked steak, fresh broccoli, and nothing else. I ate it and went right back to Gail's and to bed. The next morning: no change. Oh, well. It had been worth a try.

I got to Chris about 10:00. Georgia had arrived a little earlier with a wonderful surprise. In her class the previous day each of the children had done an "acrostic," a paper where they spelled "Christine" vertically on the left side of the sheet and then used each letter of her name to begin a sentence or sentiment about her. Since Georgia had told them about Chris's cancer, and the children had met her when we visited the school earlier that week, they were interested to hear about her progress in the hospital. The acrostics were intended to help Chris feel better, and they were decorated with colorful drawings. Some of the children even attached photos of themselves in the form of little stickers. Each paper was mounted on a somewhat larger piece of heavy construction paper, creating the effect that they were matted. They were sweet, funny, and touching, and it really brightened up the room when Georgia taped them up on the walls.

Just after lunch, a very large physical therapist arrived to take Chris on another "walk." This woman was very nice, all 300 pounds of her. Chris was so weak that this woman had trouble getting her out of bed, but she did and they walked a few steps after which Chris sat down on a chair that had wheels. Big mistake. The chair started to roll backwards as Chris was lowering herself into it and she got a scare, which caused her to tense up which is not a fun feeling to have when you have a new incision across your abdomen from hip to hip. She did land in the chair, but the stress of the moment caused Chris to start having a hypoglycemic shock episode and we all rushed in to give her some sugar and keep her from falling out of the chair.

In the process of this excitement, her gown came down exposing the dressings on her "new" breast and I yelled out, "Oh, my God! Your nipple fell off!"

That sort of broke the tension and we all chuckled. Chris stayed in the chair for a few minutes and then got back into bed, pretty much spent for the rest of the day.

The next day, Sunday, I awoke and as soon as my feet touched the floor I noticed that the middle toe on my right foot was sore. It was actually pretty shocking; the day before there was nothing wrong, but today it hurt like hell. It was red and swollen, too. I figured that maybe I had stubbed it in the middle of the night on my way to the bathroom and didn't remember, because there was no other explanation for it. I could think of nothing that had happened recently that could have caused such a thing. I thought it would go away as I got going for the day. It didn't.

By the time I got to Chris's bedside I had a noticeable limp; it was really painful! I didn't feel that I could complain, though, with my wife lying there all stitched up. The discomfort changed from hour to hour, and sometimes I even forgot about it.

I was disappointed to find out that I had missed a visit from the occupational therapist, who had gotten Chris out of bed and helped her walk down the hall and back. Chris was feeling pretty good about it. She and the therapist had been walking slowly down the hall; Chris didn't know how fast she was supposed to go. Then the therapist said, "Can't you walk any faster?" and Chris picked up the pace. She was slightly bent because of the abdominal incision so the therapist said, "Can't you straighten up any?"

Chris just stopped and stared at her with a twinkle in her eye. "Don't you *know* what kind of surgery I just had?"

Later that afternoon a big moment arrived, a moment about which I had been asking the nurses for *hours*. As soon as we had had a surgery date, I inquired about having a therapy dog come to visit Chris while she was in the hospital. This is a wonderful program where specially trained dogs are allowed in to see the patients who want to see them (with medical clearance, of course). The bond between people and animals is very strong and studies have shown that such contact has a calming and therefore healing affect on the patients. One of Chris's concerns about the whole hospital-thing was being away from her animals for so long, so I thought that this would be a wonderful thing for her. I was right.

From her first day there I inquired about a therapy dog visit and was told that they usually come on Sundays; it was Sunday and I was asking about it every hour or so. I had wanted it to be a surprise, but had neglected to tell the hospital staff that little fact, so someone had already mentioned it to Chris before the dog finally got there. There's an important lesson: if you want to surprise someone with something, be sure that everyone who could potentially spoil the surprise knows not to let the cat out of the bag!

The dog arrived and Chris lit up like a Christmas tree. It was a little dog, a Schipperke named "Kodiak" complete with her very own little hospital photo-ID tag (just like the doctors' and nurses') hanging on the little collar around her little neck. She was very sweet and her owner put her on the bed so Chris could pet her.

Chris and Kodiak had a lovely visit for about 15 minutes, and we took lots of photos. It was a wonderful experience that I highly recommend for anyone who loves animals.

Later that day Chris went on another walk, which I watched with great pride. Since she was able to walk on her own, they removed the catheter since she would now be able to get to the bathroom. Chris was a bit disappointed, though, because she thought it was "groovy" that she never had to get out of bed to go to the bathroom!

My toe got worse as the day progressed, and Chris started insisting that I have someone look at it. After all, she told me, one of the best emergency rooms in the world was right downstairs! About 9:00 p.m. I decided she was probably right, so I went to Emergency and several doctors looked at my foot and decided that the problem was caused by an infection so they prescribed some antibiotics. They had ruled out gout because of the location and color of the swelling. While I was in there, I had them look at my throat as well to make sure it wasn't strep throat or anything more serious than a common cold. It wasn't. In the course of admitting me into the E/R, I got a little ID bracelet just like Chris's, although it was a different color.

I got back to Chris's room about 11:00 p.m. and she was watching the news on TV. She had been very concerned so I told her what happened and said, "I may have a cold and a really sore toe, but my nipples are both okay!" She laughed, but then she usually does; she is my best audience. I proudly showed her my bracelet.

"Look! Just like yours!"

She held up her wrist and we put our bracelets side by side and admired them facetiously, cocking our heads in mock adoration of this wonderful bond between us. It was so silly we laughed out loud and we were having fun, despite the bizarre circumstance in which we found ourselves. I cannot

---

"I cannot overemphasize the importance of . . . finding humor in the situation, no matter how unpleasant that situation may be."

---

over-emphasize the importance of being silly and finding humor in the situation, no matter how unpleasant that situation may be.

Then she told me the big news: she had gotten out of bed and gone to the bathroom *by herself!* It had been pretty painful as I'm sure you can imagine, but she toughed it out and did it. What a gal! From all indications she would be going home the next day, and this was a very good sign.

I left her about 11:30 and went to find an all-night pharmacy to get my antibiotics. Tomorrow was going to be a big day and I needed all the help I could get.

June 17:
Coming Home

The next morning my cold was going strong, my toe was painful, and I couldn't have been happier; Chris was coming home! When I walked into her room she looked very happy, and the doctors had already been there to discharge her. She was wearing her new cream-colored silk pajamas, which were perfect for the occasion.

The nurse went over her discharge instructions with me, including a prescription for a painkiller and some other things she was supposed to take. There was a post-operative appointment with Dr. Da Lio the following Monday as well.

One of our favorite nurses on Chris's floor was Rosa, an energetic and cheerful lady from Guatemala. She was always full of life with a take-no-prisoners attitude, and happy to help us with anything we needed, ending many of her sentences in her Guatemalan accent with "my darling:" "I'd be happy to do that, my darling," or "Would you like more juice, my darling?"

When I arrived in the room my toe was particularly painful and she noticed right away. "Why are you limping, my darling?"

When I told her about my toe, she told me that she had a remedy from the ancient Mayan culture in her country. "Fill a small tub with water as hot as you can stand it, add one cup of vinegar and one tablespoon of fresh oregano, and soak your foot in it until the water cools. Repeat this as often as you like, my darling."

Uh-huh.

Although I was skeptical, it was worth a try; after all, the ancient cultures certainly had a way with mysterious cures, didn't they?

"Here is my home phone number," she said, writing it down on a piece of paper. "You call me any time if you need anything, my darling."

She was so cute; Chris and I just loved her.

"Transportation" arrived, (read that as "wheelchair") and we said goodbye to everyone and made our way down to the car. All my worries from that first lunch at the hospital were now ready to be realized... would they be? I wondered about that as I went to get the car while Chris waited at the door.

First of all, Chris was able to get into the car without too much difficulty. She is not prone to complaining and, although it was painful, she got right in and made herself comfortable. I asked if she wanted to lie down in the back, but she wanted to ride up front.

And we were off!

At first I flinched at every bump, concerned that any jarring, no matter how small, would hurt her. It didn't. Everything was going smoothly for the first hour or so as we cruised down the freeway, each of us on a cell phone calling friends and family to tell them the good news. Then Chris needed to make a bathroom stop. She is partial to Chevron stations, so I saw one in the distance and exited the freeway.

I went in to make sure that the bathroom wasn't occupied before Chris made the journey in. Surprise! The mini-mart was attached to a McDonald's restaurant, and they shared the bathroom! This meant that Chris had to walk, in her silk pajamas, hair unwashed for five days, and no make-up, through a crowded McDonald's to get to the bathroom. Sure, why not?

I went back to the car and told Chris the situation. She was pretty resigned to the whole scene and said, philosophically, "Sometimes ya just gotta do what ya gotta do!"

I helped her out of the car and we were quite a sight as she shuffled gingerly, awkwardly, and v e r y s l o w l y through the restaurant while I held on to her for dear life. I deposited her in the bathroom and waited patiently outside until she reappeared, and then we repeated our little parade in reverse.

We hit the road again but were getting hungry, so we stopped at In 'n Out Burger, a drive thru restaurant that we like but rarely allow ourselves to enjoy because of health issues. As we waited in the drive-thru line Chris decided that she wanted to get in the back seat to lie down after we ate, so we both got out of the car (in the drive-thru line) and I helped her get out of the front and into the back. I got back in and then proceeded through the line to get our food. I'm sure that was quite a sight as well, with her in her silk pajamas, etc.

We made it home safely and without further incident, not even a traffic stop for a carpool lane violation! Once again my worries about getting home were unfounded, once again proving the value of the "Don't-go-there-'til-you-get-there" philosophy.

Before we arrived, I called Kate to make sure that she had the dogs contained so we could get into the house without being joyously greeted. Once home, Chris settled into a comfy chair with pillows protecting her dressings and we let the dogs in to see her one at a time. After the initial hysteria was over, I helped her into bed with the remote controls for the TV and VCR, as well as one of the walkie-talkie radios, and she went right to sleep.

The next order of business was to get the prescriptions filled, so I went to our pharmacy and took care of that while Chris slept so she would have her pain medication when she needed it.

Later that night I was hobbling around like a 90-year-old man trying to get Chris comfortable, get both of us some dinner, and take care of all the animals. I couldn't believe how much I used that darned toe, and it was REALLY uncomfortable. When I was finished with my chores for the day, I figured I had nothing to lose so I made the concoction of water, vinegar, and oregano that Rosa had told me about and soaked my foot in it: it felt better immediately and was virtually pain-free. Amazing.

At 7:00 the next morning I found Chris outside gingerly shuffling down the driveway with a fistful of carrots, inspecting her flower garden on her way to visit with the horses. The barn is about 20 feet lower than the house and there is a sloped area to walk down to get there, but the horses' area comes all the way up to a portion of the driveway, which is level with the entrance to the house. I walked with her to the end of the driveway where she could visit with the horses through the fence with no steep inclines. They were happy to see her and she them as well.

And there she was, surrounded by dogs and horses in our little piece of heaven; the best medicine for her, that's for sure!

Later that day she had her first shower since the morning of the surgery, including a wash, dry, and style of her hair. She felt a whole lot better after that, as I'm sure you can imagine.

Also that day, Tuesday, Dr. Brooks called to tell us that the pathology report showed "clean margins" all around, which meant that it was highly unlikely that any of the tumor still remained... they got it all! She is so sweet and kind; she sounded almost as happy about it as we were! This was what Dr. Loman had hoped to do but could not within the scope of the procedure that he had performed. He had done a wonderful job, but the tumor had been just too large to be removed in a lumpectomy.

The next few days were much like the days after the lumpectomy, with a few new twists. For one, Chris could not use her abdominal muscles because of the incision, so we worked out a system where I could help her when she needed it. When getting out of a chair, for example, I held out my hand so she could use it as an anchor, pulling against it. I held it steady for her without pulling so that she had total control of her progress. If I pulled too hard or too fast she could get hurt, so doing it this way worked very well.

Our experience after the lumpectomy served us well, although everything we did before had to be done in light of much more serious incisions and dressings. And four, count 'em, FOUR drains to empty and keep track of instead of just one.

My post-operative duties included changing some of the surgical dressings. Every day. They sent Chris home with her breast heavily padded with gauze and her abdominal incision covered with gauze that was held in place by an 8-inch wide elastic bandage that wrapped completely and tightly around her, stuck to itself and secured with Velcro. In order to change the dressing, I had to remove the elastic and the old, icky gauze, then replace the gauze and re-fit the elastic, all without putting any pressure on the incision. Considering that the incision was from hip to hip, it was a little tricky until I got the hang of it.

It wasn't too bad as long as I didn't think about them telling me that the elastic around Chris's waist was "holding her together;" I envisioned a scene right out of the movie "Alien," when an alien burst out of the chest of one of the astronauts during dinner on the spaceship. Chris just wasn't ready to look at the incisions, so I got the first peek. I must say that even I was a bit squeamish at first because it looked pretty raw, and sometimes the gauze was stuck and I was afraid of hurting her when I removed it. I didn't blame her for not wanting to look, and I played it down so she wouldn't freak-out more than she already was.

Showering was pretty much the same, except Chris had to sit on the little bench that we have in the shower. I bathed Chris gingerly, using the showerhead on the long hose to carefully direct the water away from the areas that were supposed to stay dry.

In order to wash her hair, once again Chris had to lie on the kitchen counter which was a nearly impossible task considering her gargantuan abdominal incision. It had been much easier after the lumpectomy because the incisions were much smaller. Making the situation more difficult was the fact that the counter was just barely long enough for her torso, and the desired position for washing her hair required her legs to be straight up and against the cupboards. Helping her get into that position in her condition wasn't easy, but she was tough and I supported her back and head as she laid down; it was quite a scene. I positioned a rolled-up towel under her neck and she was fairly comfortable once she got in position. I confess that I took advantage of the situation and kissed her all over her face as we waited the required three minutes for the crème rinse to set. I never heard her complain about it, though, so I guess it was okay.

One problem that we hadn't thought about was *getting her back off of the counter after her hair was washed*. We didn't have too much time to figure it out because her legs, being vertical, were beginning to fall asleep so I lifted her shoulders and she pivoted around and presto!, she was sitting upright on the counter. After the initial moments of concern, it turned out to be much easier than getting her onto the counter in the first place!

It was simply amazing how few pain pills Chris took. She says that she hates taking pills and, besides, if you are always taking pain pills how do you know when you don't need them any more? That philosophy, combined with her exceptional courage and tolerance for pain, carried the day. It was very impressive.

It was virtually impossible to do everything that had to be done around the house as well as get any work done in my office. Kate, as usual, was a tremendous help. We had recognized long before the surgery that Chris wouldn't be able to ride the horses at all for at least six weeks following the surgery, and only sporadically for the next 18 weeks during chemotherapy treatments. This wasn't only sad for Chris, but unhealthy for the horses who needed to be exercised regularly. Kate jumped in and offered to ride the horses twice a week; she had a number of friends who were accomplished riders and could ride with her in turns.

Naturally, the friends were thrilled to be able to go horseback riding so it worked out well for everyone. Kate was in charge of this operation; for approximately *five months* (June through October) she scheduled and coordinated everything beautifully, and took good care of Chris's "babies." It was a great help to both of us; Chris didn't have to worry because she knew the horses were in capable hands and that they were getting the exercise they needed, and I was often relieved of some of my horse-related chores because when Kate and her friends went riding, they picked up the manure and often fed them as well. As we always say, "Kate is great!"

There was still one hellava lot to do. The morning ritual went something like this: get up, check on Chris (she was usually still asleep), walk the dogs in the forest, feed the horses, pick up the horse manure in the yard (when Kate didn't do it), feed the dogs, cats, and fish, check on Chris again, make breakfast for myself, water the flower garden in the front, water the plants on the deck, check on Chris again who was usually awake by now, make her breakfast, do the dishes, uncover Poncho, change his water, remove any dirty papers from the cage bottom, empty Chris's drains, and then, hopefully, get downstairs to the office for a half hour or so. Then it was time to take the dogs out, make lunch for the two of us, eat, do the dishes, walk down to the barn and give the horses some hay, and so on.

Afternoons were usually a good time to give the girl her shower and wash and dry her hair. Then, perhaps, I would have a little time to try to get something done before the evening chores began: water the flower garden again (if it had been hot), walk the dogs, feed the horses, make dinner for the two of us, eat, do the dishes… sheesh, I'm getting tired just writing all of this! We usually spent time together in the evening, but then the evening chores kicked in; empty Chris's

> "It's too easy to get caught in the trap of feeling like the current situation is permanent, resulting in a feeling of overwhelming hopelessness."

drains, cut up carrots for the horses, change Poncho's dirty papers and water, cover his cage, take the dogs out, and go down to the barn to give the horses their carrots, hay, and evening supplements. Bedtime for me those days was usually between midnight and 1:00 a.m. I always knew that Chris did a lot around the house, but I had an entirely fresh appreciation for just how much that was.

As each day wore on I found myself, once again, getting discouraged, overwhelmed, and afraid. Not only for Chris and what would happen to her, although I never really thought she would die, but mainly the money situation, which wasn't getting any better. The later it was in the day, the more upset I got, and it was a never-ending cycle. Added to the mix was a bad case of "cabin fever," a feeling that I was stuck in the house and couldn't go anywhere without feeling guilty about it. I could go from elation to despair and back again in a five-minute period, depending on what was going on.

I always enjoyed being around Chris and helping her, and those were the high points of the day. But the chores and responsibilities were just too much to think about and left me with no time to make any money; the frustration level was, at times, unbearable. The only way I could deal with it was to not deal with it at all, realizing that this was just something that I had to get through and that it was only temporary. It's one thing to know that intellectually, but another to actually *feel* it, and I had to keep reminding myself in order to maintain my sanity. It's too easy to get caught in the trap of feeling like the current situation is permanent, resulting in a feeling of overwhelming hopelessness. It takes an ongoing, concerted effort to contain those feelings and to keep yourself aware of the fact that this new and unpleasant reality is only temporary.

The drains were much more of an issue with this surgery than the last because there were four of them instead of just one; four drains to empty and keep track of, four drains to protect from water and damage, and four drains to carefully attach (with safety pins) to everything she wore. After my experience with the first drain I was more skilled at dealing with them than before.

Or was I?

I numbered the drains 1 – 4 so I could keep track of the amount of fluid produced by each one. I had to empty them twice a day, so "Oh! Canada" rang through the house often. Part of the ritual included "milking" the drains if they seemed to need it. I was a little nervous about that so I asked our neighbor, Kathy the E.R. nurse, to come over and show me how. At the time Kathy was able to come over, Chris and I were in the barn, so the horses got to learn how to milk the drains right along with me!

Kathy showed me how to pinch the tube about an inch from where it emerged from Chris and hold it steady while pinching the tube with my other hand and then "sliding the pinch" toward the bulb in order to dislodge anything that was stuck in the tube. In the process of sliding the pinch, the tube would stretch between my two hands, but the tube could not be pulled outward from Chris's body because of the hand that was holding it steady; the mere thought of that gave us both the heebie-jeebies.

Everything was going well as the days passed and I was getting to feel pretty good about my newfound drain-handling abilities when I made what turned out to be a big boo-boo. In the process of "sliding the pinch" down the tube, I acciden-tally moved my other hand, which resulted in the tube being pulled outward from Chris. Since the tube was held in place by a stitch that went around the tube and then through Chris's skin, it pulled on that stitch and Chris yelped. Naturally, I felt terrible that I had hurt her and we both became gun-shy about milking any more drains, but I was much more careful after that and didn't repeat that particular error.

The damage had been done, however, and the net result was that the tube had apparently been pulled out just enough to cause constant pulling on the stitch that was holding it in place. It was the drain on the side of her reconstructed breast and it felt to Chris like a thorn was stuck in her skin. What had I done? I was mortified. At first I was hoping that it was just sore from the unintentional yanking it got, but the next day it still hurt her and, at 11:45 Saturday night she woke me up and said it hurt so much she couldn't sleep.

I figured that the only way to fix it would be to cut the stitch, thereby relieving the pulling on her skin. But if I did that, what would hold the tube in place? We were going for our post-operative appointment the following Monday; if I snipped the stitch now would it be okay until then?

At this point we had been home five full days and that particular drain was not producing much fluid, so I came to the horrifying conclusion that the drain was going to have to be pulled out and that I was probably going to have to do it.

I wasn't about to do anything that dramatic without some guidance, so I paged the plastic surgeon that was on-call and we waited. About 30 minutes later he called back. I explained the situation and he agreed that the stitch had to be cut, and that definitely meant that the drain would have to come out because we could not leave it in without the stitch there to hold it in place. I told him the amount of fluid that the drain was producing and he said that it was time for the drain to come out anyway, so it wouldn't be a problem.

Right. Not for *him*!

He told me to remove the cap from the bulb and empty the bulb like I always did, but to leave the cap off so there would be no suction applied to the end of the tube that I was pulling. Otherwise it would be harder to pull, be much more painful for Chris, and could cause some damage on the way out.

What about the hole that it leaves? Is it going to bleed like crazy? How do I patch it up?

I was *way* outside my comfort zone.

He told me that it probably wouldn't bleed much, and to just put a bandage over it.

How much tubing will come out? I was imagining three feet of tubing with blood and entrails attached... what the hell was I doing in this situation??

He said that it would only be about five or six inches. I told him my fears and tried to make light of it and he assured me that it would all be okay, and we laughed about it together. Sort-of.

I remember thinking, "Am I really having this conversation? It's midnight; is this simply a nightmare?" I even started to calculate how difficult it would be to drive to UCLA, but getting dressed and ready to go, followed by two hours in each direction was just too much. And what about the animals? We could go to our local hospital, but Chris said she had confidence in me and didn't want to leave the house.

So...

Chris immediately took one of her pain pills even though she wasn't "due" for one. We went into the bathroom and she sat on the edge of the tub. I knew that we better do this right away because the more I thought about it, the more freaked-out I got. I can only imagine how Chris felt, but she was very brave (as she had been about everything else) and trusted me completely. We looked at each other and laughed nervously at the situation in which we found ourselves. Chris said, "Now listen, 'Nurse Dave'. Just promise me that you won't run screaming from the room until after it's completely out!" That helped to break the tension a bit.

First, I cut the stitch and her thorn-like discomfort stopped immediately. I pulled out the little threads from the stitch: so far, so good. Then I emptied the bulb and we sang

"It's surprising what you're capable of doing when you have to."

"Oh! Canada," with trembling voices at the thought of what we were about to do. Leaving the cap off of the bulb as instructed, I was ready to pull it out. Then I told her to take a few deep, cleansing, relaxing breaths; I don't know why, it just seemed like a good idea.

We took them together. One, two, THREE... and I pulled. At first, there was some resistance and the thought went through my mind that I hadn't relieved the suction properly, but once the tube started to move it was out in a flash. As predicted, only about six inches came out and, happily, there were no entrails attached. There was no blood either, just a hole in Chris's side. It was weird.

As I pulled, Chris had made a grunting noise, more to mask the pain than to express it. She said it hurt, but only for a second and then it was okay.

I held up the drain like a trophy and I became overwhelmed with relief that it was over and that it was okay. It was almost 1:30 in the morning, so being tired didn't help. We complimented each other on our bravery and Chris gave me a big hug and thanked me.

It's surprising what you're capable of doing when you have to.

I experienced a feeling that I don't recall ever having before; a combination of relief, pride, renewed self-confidence, and that incredible satisfaction knowing that I was taking good care of Chris. It was quite a rush.

I put a bandage over the hole left by the drain and we went back to bed.

June 24:
The Post-Op Appointment

After the excitement of "The Drain Incident" Saturday night, Sunday turned out to be pretty boring! The day after that, however, was the post-op appointment with Dr. Da Lio. Chris was feeling pretty good and was easily walking around the house so we left early to go to Costco. We didn't think it would be wise for her to do more walking than she had to, so she used one of their electric carts with a shopping basket attached. We agreed to meet near the pharmacy and off she went, disappearing into the cavernous store.

After I got what I needed I started looking for her and, turning the corner there she was, her little smiling face just barely visible above a huge pile of stuff she had managed to get into the basket, toodling down the aisle toward me. I laughed out loud; she was so darned cute! As it turned out, she had had several encounters with very nice people who were anxious to help her, one of whom said, "If you need any help, just ask. People want to help you!" Later, she "motored" over to the bathroom and they let her go to the front of the line. The whole experience was wonderful, and we came away with a good feeling about how kind people can be.

The appointment with Dr. Da Lio was a little scary because we knew that they would probably remove the remaining three drains. The nurse was very impressed that I had removed the one drain, and congratulated me on my courage. The drains were out before we knew it, each of which hurt Chris like hell, but for only a second.

The doctor came in and inspected his work with pride. He took off the dressings and the new breast was impressive-looking, that's for sure. There was a smooth patch of skin where her areola and nipple used to be, both of which had been removed because of the cancer. Basically, in layman's terms, the surgeons removed the areola and nipple, scooped out the cancerous tissue through the opening, and then inserted the tissue from her abdomen. Then they "patched" the hole with some of the skin that had been removed when the abdominal tissue was harvested. Obviously, that is outrageously understated and simplified but, in concept, it is accurate. The patch would later be molded into a nipple in the second stage of the reconstruction, and then, finally, tattooed to match the areola of the other breast.

I asked Dr. Da Lio when the second stage of the reconstruction would be and he said that he likes to do it between the end of chemotherapy and the beginning of radiation. It is a simple, outpatient procedure and Chris would be pretty much back to normal within two days. Plus, he would need to see her before they could schedule the surgery.

I immediately realized how much advance planning and coordination it was going to take to make that happen, because of lead times to get an appointment and all of the resources he would need for the surgery; team, operating room, anesthesiologist, recovery, etc. Not to mention coordinating with the schedule for radiation. "Don't go there 'til you get there" was running through my head and I decided not to worry about it until the next-to-last chemo treatment, whenever that was going to be.

I asked the doctor how long we had to wait to schedule chemotherapy and he said that, as far as he was concerned, three weeks from the date of the surgery Chris would be considered "healed" and could do just about anything she felt like doing. The only exception was that she should wear the elastic bandage to support her abdomen for six weeks.

The next day I scheduled the chemotherapy consult for July 9. The three-week anniversary of the surgery was the Fourth of July, so the 9th was pretty close.

June 25:
The Midnight Ride

Later that evening Chris was complaining that the tissue in her reconstructed breast seemed to be getting more and more firm as the day went on. I felt it and it seemed to me to be as hard as a rock, and very heavy. I didn't remember it being that hard to the touch, so I called the plastic surgeon on call. I told him about it and he asked several questions, then told us he would call us back in about an hour; he felt that they should take a look at it because the area may be bleeding internally in which case they would have to go in and repair the area.

Oh-oh. It was about 10:00 p.m. and we're talking about a two-hour drive. We started preparing for an all-nighter and, perhaps, another hospital stay.

When the surgeon called back he told us that we should come in, that he wanted to take a look at it. I looked at the clock: 10:45. The first thing I did, as much as I hated to do it, was call Kate because we were going to be gone all night plus who knows how long the next day and the animals had to be taken care of. I knew that Kate normally went to bed around 10:00, so I was afraid that I would be waking her up. I was. She very sleepily said that she'd be right over; "Kate is great!"

Chris and I then frantically tried to think of everything we would need and loaded up the car. Kate had sounded pretty sleepy and, frankly, I was afraid that she would fall back to sleep, but about 11:15 she pulled up in her car still dressed in her pajamas, said "Hello" in a sleepy voice, and disappeared into the house. Geez, how we love that woman!

We left the house at 11:30 and got to the bottom of the mountain at midnight, at which time Chris had to make a restroom stop. At first they didn't want to let her into the mini-mart, which was locked at night, but fortunately it was a woman at the register and when Chris told her her story and what we were doing, the woman let her right in. I figured I might as well get gas while I was waiting, and casually looked in the back of the 4Runner while it was filling up. Something was missing. My bag. My toiletries. My change of clothes. Some bad words were said, and I bought a bottle of Mountain Dew because I didn't know of any other drink that had more caffeine; I figured this was going to be an even longer night that I had thought.

So we drove back up the mountain, picked up the bag, and left the house for the second time at 12:30 a.m.

The drive was uneventful. The excitement of the adventure (and the Mountain Dew) kept me awake, Chris slept in the back, and we didn't need to use the carpool lane. There wasn't much traffic, but I couldn't help but wonder why the people who *were* on the road were driving around at such a horrible hour.

We arrived at the emergency room about 2:15 a.m. on Wednesday morning and, as we walked in, couldn't help but notice a woman who looked homeless who was ranting and raving although we couldn't tell what about. Two uniformed policemen, who had apparently just brought her in, were waiting for some paperwork before leaving. When I saw them there I thought to myself this might be a perfect opportunity to ask them about driving in the carpool lane with Chris sleeping in the back: what should I do if I saw the dreaded flashing lights in my rearview mirror?

We had paged the surgeon on call from the car about 20 minutes before we arrived, and we went through the check-in procedure, getting registered and moving into a treatment room. While Chris was getting checked in I approached the officers and told them my dilemma.

"My wife has breast cancer and we drive 2 hours each way to get her treatments. She lies down in the back and sleeps on the way so it looks like I'm alone in the car, but I use the carpool lane. First of all, am I allowed to use it and secondly, what should I do if I get pulled over? Should I have her stick an arm or leg out the window so the officer can see that I am not alone in the car?"

I can't give you their exact answer, but the gist of it was yes, I can use the carpool lane and if I were to get pulled over I should just move to the right shoulder as soon as it is safe to do so. When the officer sees that Chris is in the car sleeping, they will tell me to have a nice day and be on my way, unless, of course, they were pulling me over for some other reason! The requirement for using the carpool lane, they told me, is that two or more people have to be *in* the car, not necessarily *visible* in the car.

I thanked them and went back to Chris. For some reason I find it intimidating to talk to uniformed policemen perhaps because, fortunately, I haven't had occasion to deal with them much for any reason thus far in my life. I sure do respect them and the courage that they must have just to do their job on a day-to-day basis. Can you imagine pulling a car over and approaching complete strangers to tell them they've done something wrong? How much courage does *that* take?

I was reminded of being at my sister's apartment in New York City about six weeks after the September 11 attacks. A gas leak had been reported in front of her building and about 20 firemen arrived complete with sirens and flashing lights. After all I had seen on television related to the attacks and the heroic efforts of the New York Fire Department, seeing them up close and personal was somewhat overwhelming when I had gone to the street to see what was going on.

Talking with those officers left me with that same "they are larger-than-life" feeling of awe and respect.

The on-call doctor told us that Chris shouldn't eat anything after midnight in the event that they had to do more surgery, but I was hungry so after Chris was situated in the treatment room I went to the vending machine that I had found the previous week when I was there for my toe. When I returned, the doctor had just arrived and he took a look at the reconstruction and seemed unsure about the firmness. He wanted to have Dr. Da Lio look at it and decided to call him about 6:00 a.m. I looked at my watch: 3:30. 2 ½ hours to wait in that little room. Fortunately, Chris was on a gurney and was comfy with a blanket and pillow, so she was asleep in no time. I, on the other hand, had only a plastic chair.

All my life I have been fortunate in that I can sleep just about anywhere. I distinctly remember being on a school bus in the 7th grade on the way back from a school outing to the opera. It was bouncy and noisy, not only from the bus and traffic but from 30 other kids talking and yelling. I not only fell asleep, I slept for almost the entire hour back to school! I can doze off while waiting for a movie to start, and a five-minute catnap makes me feel like a new person. So I wasn't worried about being able to sleep in that uncomfortable little chair, but considering how tired I was and how much sleep I needed, this was going to be a challenge even for me.

I sat there, chin against my chest, dozing on and off for the entire 2 ½ hours. I could hear Chris's heavy breathing so I knew that she was getting some good sack time, but I was not. Every now and then she woke up and was very thirsty, just as she had been immediately after the surgery, so I went looking for ice chips to give her.

Six o'clock came and went with no word. At about 7:00 I went upstairs to the "TRAM-flap unit" to see if I could find anyone who could tell me what was going on. I encountered the plastic surgery residents (but not Dr. Da Lio) as they were making their rounds checking on patients. They told me that they knew about Chris in the emergency room and would be down to see her in about 30 minutes.

Sure enough, at 7:30 they all arrived, examined Chris, and decided to admit her to the hospital. Gulp. Was she really going to have to have surgery again? Although this had been discussed since 11:00 the night before, it was scarier now that it seemed more definite.

Again we waited, this time for an admitting person to come in to do the paperwork and for Chris to be assigned to a room. It was about 9:00 when they finally came to move her to a room on the same floor where she had been before. It was like old-home week as we greeted everyone and they were happy to see us, although not under the circumstances.

About 9:45, Dr. Da Lio arrived. He had been surprised to hear that we were there, having just seen Chris two days earlier when everything seemed okay. He looked at the reconstruction, palpated it (medical mumbo-jumbo for "pressed it a few times with his fingers") and said, "There's nothing wrong with this."

WHAT??

He continued. "It's the same as it was on Monday; I told you then that it would feel hard like this for a while as blood accumulated, but that it would return to normal in a month or two." He wasn't angry or even slightly annoyed, just very matter-of-fact. "Go home. You're fine." He smiled at us, we thanked him, and he was gone.

We were stunned. We spent all night there for no reason? I wasn't mad, just frustrated. Given the same circumstances I would have done it again in a second; it was really the only thing we *could* have done. But still…

Chris got dressed, we signed some papers, and we were on our way. Chris hadn't been able to eat anything in preparation for a possible surgery, so she was hungry and so was I. We decided to go to Junior's, a wonderful delicatessen we had tried after one of Chris's other appointments.

Naturally, when you are as hungry as we were, you order much more than you can eat and we definitely did. We both had a craving for onion rings but they always gross us out after we've eaten just a few, so we got a half-order along with some sandwiches. The half-order was still about 3 times as much as we wanted, so we each had only two. When we left, Chris took the leftover onion rings over to two complete strangers and asked if they wanted them! She assured them that we had only eaten a couple and, other than that, they were untouched. They accepted with a big smile.

The drive home was not uneventful. It was almost noon and I was much too tired to be driving. We could have gone to Gail's to get some sleep, but that would have resulted in having to drive home either during the rush hour traffic or after it; neither scenario was particularly appealing to us. So I thought I'd tough it out.

Big mistake.

It only took about 20 minutes before I was fighting the fatigue. Chris still wasn't supposed to drive and was sleeping in the back. I was jumping around in the seat, air conditioning on full blast to keep myself as cold as possible, rubbing my head; in retrospect it was just plain stupid.

About half way home I guess I dozed off while driving because I was startled by the horn blast of an eighteen-wheeler after I apparently drifted over into his lane. That was it. I was scared into submission and I immediately got off the freeway to collect myself. It was pretty warm outside and there was no way I could sleep without some shade. I realized that there was a mall with covered parking about two freeway exits away, so I decided that I would just have to make it. I did, we parked under cover, and I slept for about 45 minutes. It wasn't much, but it was enough to get us home without further incident.

About a week later, in an effort to help other women in our community, Chris wrote the following letter to the editor of our local newspaper.

> *April 10th I was taking my evening shower when I felt a lump in my breast. I told myself it's probably just a cyst and I went to see Dr. Win the next day. After a mammogram and a biopsy, Dr. Win called us into her office at 8pm on our wedding anniversary. I knew that couldn't be good. My husband, Dave, was by my side as she told us, "You have breast cancer".*

At that moment, I looked at the clock; not only was it our anniversary, but it was the exact time we were married as well.

Dr. Win prayed with us and for all of the doctors and nurses that would be entering into our lives, and wished us good luck.

I know that none of us get out of here alive: something will get us all in the end, but I've always tried to do the best for my body and eat wisely. No fatty foods, lots of dark green vegetables, no dairy, and lots of fish and dark red berries. I read two health magazines and take many vitamins and herbal supplements in order to prevent cancer.

There has never been any cancer in my family of any kind, let alone breast caner. My ancestors all lived into their 80's and 90's.

I always go for a physical and mammogram every year, and every year I've gotten a clean bill of health. As it turns out, a mammogram only seven months earlier showed no sign of the tumor: breast cancer is commonly in your body for many years before it shows its ugly head. Doctors, friends, and family are at a loss as to "why me". Stuff happens, I guess.

The reason I'm sharing this is because early detection is the key to saving your life. Know your body well. Look for subtle changes, and if you don't have the same bump on each side, go see your physician immediately!

Since I found it relatively early, I've been given a 70% chance of living five years by the Revlon/UCLA Breast Center. (Another hospital said it was a 50% - 60% chance.) At UCLA, which is one of the top-rated breast cancer centers in the country, I feel like they put a warm blanket around me each time I'm there. It has been a wonderful experience for both my hus-

*husband and me and, in many ways, it has actually
been a gift. The only bad thing for me has been that
my very physical life has stopped; but I know it's
only temporary.*

*I have a fantastic husband who loves me too
much, so I don't know how I'd be without him by
my side. (When this all started, I told him, "On the
roller coaster of life, it's our turn to sit in the front
car.") Family, neighbors, and great friends have also
been a tremendous help.*

*I will probably continue to eat salmon and broc-
coli for breakfast, but I'm going to have pie now
whenever I want.*

Christine Balch

July 1 was Chris's 50th birthday, so Gail and Sonia treated
us to dinner at our favorite Japanese restaurant in the city.
We had some errands to run before dinner, so we arranged to
meet them at the restaurant. We finished our errands early
and were already seated in the restaurant when, once again,
in walked a tremendous pile of wrapped gifts.

Believe it or not, there were 50 gifts, in honor of Chris's
50th. Some were small (pieces of Chris's favorite candy),
some were large (a large, beautiful wicker basket, in which
many of the gifts had been festively arranged), but there were
50 of them nonetheless, including a new zoom-lens camera.
Gail and Sonia are simply amazing; is there no limit to their
generosity?

July 9:
The Chemotherapy Consult

Two weeks passed and Chris got better each day. She began to resume her usual activities as quickly as she could; she didn't like the fact that I had to take care of so many of her responsibilities.

July 9th arrived and we made the 2-hour trip to Dr. Chap's office, which was part of UCLA but in a different location. As it turned out, it was almost exactly the same mileage for us even though it was about six miles from the hospital and Revlon/UCLA Breast Center.

Several times during the day Chris asked me, "Now tell me again what we're doing today?" I got a little cranky and began to resent the fact that I was making all of the appointments and worrying about the schedule. Once we got into the examination room, like a jerk, I commented, "Gee, it must be nice not to have to worry about any of the scheduling."

"Trade ya," she snapped back.

I felt like a complete idiot. Of course she was right; what did I have to complain about? I was ashamed of myself for even entertaining such feelings.

"You're right. I'm sorry."

It was a bad moment, but it was over quickly.

Dr. Chap came into the room and the tension disappeared immediately. We told her right off the bat that we had decided not to participate in the study that her assistant had told us about at the multi-disciplinary conference, mainly because of the distances involved. We had determined that we would have to have all of our treatments closer to home, and that Chris would have to come in once a week for several months. It was just too much, even though it was closer and, besides, we wanted to come to UCLA.

With that out of the way, she told us that in Chris's situation she felt we could go for a cure rather than simply remission. She felt that we had a good chance of getting rid of the cancer completely, but we couldn't be sure for 10 years.

My left-brain self asked, out loud, "10 years from when? The surgery? The end of the chemo? When?"

Chris and Dr. Chap laughed. "10 years from the date of the diagnosis," she told me. "At 3 years we celebrate, at 5 we have a party, and at 10 years we dance on the ceiling."

She said that there were two types of chemo that were appropriate for Chris's situation, and that Chris could choose. One of them was stronger than the other and would be harder on her, but would only be six treatments as opposed to eight treatments for the lesser-strength regimen.

Chris immediately, without giving it a second thought, said she wanted the stronger treatment not only to have the best chance of knocking out the cancer, but to get it over with as soon as possible. If it was harder, so be it; she wanted what was best for her medically and to hell with how hard it would be.

Good for you, Chris! What a brave girl!

Dr. Chap agreed but said she wanted to offer both treatments just the same.

She explained the situation to us. Now that the tumor itself was gone, the concern was that the cancer had spread to other parts of her body. The fact that Chris had six of 14 lymph nodes test positive told them that some of the cancer cells had escaped into her lymph system before the tumor was removed. If the cancer cells were circulating in her body, then they could take hold just about anywhere and begin to grow new tumors. The CT-scan (of her organs) and the bone scan (of her, uh, bones) had shown that nothing was growing at this point, but that doesn't mean that the bad guys aren't out there but too small to show up on those tests.

The treatment plan was two-fold. Once again, she explained that chemotherapy is "systemic" meaning that it treats the entire body, and radiation therapy is "local" meaning that it treats the area closest to where the tumor had been. Between the two strategies, they expected to kill any and all errant cells that were out there.

Chemotherapy would be once every three weeks for six treatments, followed by radiation therapy, which was usually five days a week, Monday through Friday, for six weeks. Dr. Chap said that she wasn't a radiologist so she wasn't 100% sure of what they would recommend, but that was usually the way it was scheduled.

I was trying to lay this all out in my mind, and wanted to know when it would all be over. At the risk of being laughed at again for my detail-oriented questions, I asked, "How long between the end of chemo and the beginning of radiation?"

"Four to six weeks."

"When is the first treatment?"

"How 'bout Friday?"

I quickly figured out a rough estimate that the radiation would be over sometime in late January or early February. Good heavens! That's a pretty long course of treatment, I thought; February seemed an awfully long time away. For insurance purposes, that wasn't too bad because most of the treatments would be in the 2002 calendar year, and subject to only that one deductible. (I know it's tacky to be thinking about money at this juncture, but it is part of my responsibility to manage the finances and it could not be ignored.)

The details of the chemo treatments were surprising. Dr. Chap told us that Chris needed to have a blood test the day before each treatment to make sure that her white blood cells were not too compromised. If they were, we would have to delay the treatment until the blood work was within acceptable limits. She was also going to give us a steroid that Chris had to take for three days, starting the day before each treatment. Then there were three different medications she was going to give us for possible nausea, which is the most common side effect of the chemo, and she explained the various combinations that she could take. (It was a good thing I had the tape recorder going... I never would have remembered all of this.)

Another effect of chemotherapy is that, in the process of killing the bad guys in the body (cancer cells) it also would kill off the good guys (white blood cells), which would leave Chris susceptible to infection. Considering the distance we had to travel, Dr. Chap was also going to give Chris an antibiotic to take for five days following each treatment as a preemptive measure. An infection could, potentially, cause her to be hospitalized.

Yes, she would lose her hair about 2 weeks after the first treatment and yes, it would definitely grow back beginning about a month after the last treatment. She gave us a prescription for a "cranial prosthesis" (a wig!) because sometimes insurance will pay for one if there is a doctor's order to get one.

Whew! That was a lot to remember!

She wrote out all of the prescriptions including one for the blood test, which we could have done at our local hospital the day before each treatment. They would then fax the results to Dr. Chap's office and before we left the house for each treatment, we would simply call to make sure that the numbers were all right. I've never seen so many prescriptions written all at one time; it was going to be a challenge to keep everything straight and give Chris the right everything at the right times, which I considered to be my responsibility.

They took the first blood test right then and there, since it was only a few days before the chemo and since it was the first treatment and the blood wouldn't be compromised by prior treatments.

We talked about it on the way home and realized that we both felt like we had taken a few steps backward in view of Dr. Chap's analysis of Chris's situation. We had felt that since the surgical margins, bone scan, and CT-scan were all clean that she was pretty much in the clear. Not so. Since cancer cells had been found in Chris's lymph nodes, that indicated that it had spread, albeit microscopically, and that these individual cells could still attach themselves somewhere and begin to grow and shed more cells. That's why the chemo was so important and there were still no guarantees.

Dr. Chap did say, however, that we were "going for a cure;" since all of the tests were clean we had a pretty good chance of that. She also said not to dance on the ceiling until the 10-year mark; that's a long time to wait, and we were both bummed.

July 12:
1st Chemotherapy Treatment

The first chemotherapy treatment was scheduled for 1:00, so we had to leave the house at 10:30. Frankly, I was nervous about the whole thing but I sure wasn't going to let Chris know that. As we were getting ready, I asked her if *she* was nervous.

"No," she told me. "I'm actually kind of excited, and I didn't sleep very well last night; it's kind of like going to medical Disneyland!"

What an attitude! I complimented her on her bravery and her brother called to wish her well. She told him the Disneyland comment and, based on her earlier roller coaster metaphor, he advised her that as the drugs were going in, she should throw her hands up in the air.

It was about that time that Lily decided to kill a bluebird and bring it in to show us. Just what we needed when we're rushing to get out of the house.

Kate arrived to work and take care of the animals for us, and finally we were on our way. It was the usual configuration: Chris slept in the back while I drove, enjoying the serenity while looking in the rearview mirror for flashing lights as I cruised in the carpool lane.

Georgia was waiting for us when we arrived, and they showed us right in to the treatment room. It was a rather large, U-shaped open space with comfy reclining chairs at little stations all around the perimeter. Each area had its own draw-curtain and table for nursing supplies, along with the IV pole and its associated pump, which was an electrical device mounted on the pole that controlled the flow of the drugs into the patient's arm. A few of the stations had a TV with a VCR, and they had a rack of popular movies and a rack of books to help the patients pass the time. As it turned out, Chris's particular regimen took about 4 hours; some patients were there even longer than that.

Chris selected one of the stations and Georgia and I pulled up chairs. Chris had brought the stuffed Saint Bernard from Melissa and Jerry plus a few small stuffed frogs as a comfort tactic, so we arranged them "just so" while waiting for the treatment to begin.

The nurse, Joan, arrived to start the IV, but it took a few "sticks" of the needle before she found a good spot. I figured that she would just place the IV in the veins at her elbow joint, which is where they normally take blood, but Joan told us that one of the drugs they give is so nasty that if any of it should escape the blood vessel at the point of the IV it could cause permanent damage to her elbow joint, and that's why she inserted the IV about midway between Chris's wrist and elbow.

Chris's regimen was called "TAC," which stood for the three drugs she would be getting: Taxotere, Adriamycin, and Cytoxan. The Taxotere and Cytoxan were administered with a "drip," which means that they were supplied in a bag that hung on the IV pole, and it dripped into the IV tube at a rate that was regulated by the pump. The Adriamycin, which was bright pink, was a "push," which means that it was supplied in a large syringe that was inserted into the IV. The nurse then manually, but very slowly, forced the drug out of the syringe and into Chris's arm. It took about five minutes to empty the syringe.

There were a few other drugs that they administered to help her cope with the TAC drugs, including some anti-nausea medication and a saline solution; it was quite a project. Even though the Adriamycin took only about five minutes, the Taxotere and Cytoxan were administered separately and took quite a bit of time. The IV pole and pump were on wheels and the pump had a battery, so when Chris had to go to the bathroom, we just unplugged the unit and she just wheeled the whole contraption in there with her.

The first treatment took the longest because they wanted to introduce the drugs slowly in case she had a bad reaction.

After the IV was in place, Joan got the Adriamycin, which was very colorful, disguising the fact that it was pretty strong stuff. It went in without a problem, and then she started the bag of Cytoxan. Georgia and I watched Chris to see if she had any reaction, but there wasn't anything noticeable and we all talked and laughed as if there was nothing out of the ordinary happening like, for example, *Chris being pumped full of poison.*

We were all getting pretty hungry and I just couldn't believe that Chris wanted any food, but she did so we asked the nurses if we could bring some food in and they said, "Sure!" They even had a list of local restaurants with menus and phone numbers, so we ordered some sandwiches from a place across the street and I went over there to get them. It was surreal to be sitting there eating while Chris was getting her chemo; all three of us were eating, talking, and laughing, having a great time. Not at all what I expected for a chemo treatment, but then I had no idea *what* to expect.

All of the drugs were dispensed and we were getting ready to go when I got a surprise: I had to give Chris an injection the next day. It seems that Dr. Chap wanted Chris to have this medication to boost her white blood count, helping her compromised immune system to be less compromised. The normal procedure is for the patient to return to the chemotherapy treatment center the day after treatment, where one of the nurses would give the injection. Since we lived so far away, though, I got to do it so we wouldn't have to make an extra trip. They gave me a box labeled "Neulasta" in a plastic zip-lock bag, surrounded by cold packs. I had to keep the Neulasta in the refrigerator until approximately 24 hours after the chemo treatment was finished, let it get to room temperature, and then give it to Chris. Joan showed me how to remove the cap, how and where to give her the injection, and how to safely dispose of the empty syringe.

The prospect of giving Chris a shot really didn't bother me because we had gone through a period when we were trying to get pregnant and I had had to give Chris a shot in her hip every day for a month. One day, when I was practicing on a grapefruit as instructed, Chris snuck up behind me and screamed just as I poked the test needle into the test grapefruit, scaring the hell out of me. We still laugh about it. The bottom line; sure, why not. Bring it on, we can handle it.

Chris was feeling great when we left about 5:30 for the underground parking garage. We were on the lowest level and there were a couple of pigeons sitting on some overhead pipes. Chris was concerned that they were trapped and couldn't find their way out, so she and Georgia shooed them toward the exit, walking up several parking levels to do it. This was a woman who had just had chemotherapy??

We hit the road and Chris felt so good and we were so hungry that we stopped to try a famous Los Angeles landmark: The Apple Pan. It was a small diner that had been there for hundreds of thousands of years (well, maybe not that long) and was famous for their apple pie. We each had a hamburger and split a piece of apple pie, a very unusual meal for us because Chris rarely eats hamburgers and I rarely eat pie. We had to try it, though, and besides, how often did we get out that way?

The ride home was the usual: her sleeping in the back, me driving in the carpool lane with one eye on the rear-view mirror.

They told us that the anti-nausea drug they had given Chris would wear off in about 24 hours, so the next morning I gave her the Compazine and Ativan combination that Dr. Chap had suggested. She was feeling okay so we decided to go to the movies. During the movie she went to the car to get a sucker, and while she was eating her sucker and popcorn one of her crowns fell out. Why not? We don't have enough to deal with, do we?

We got home and I helped her "cement in" the crown with Vaseline (as recommended by our dentist), and I gave her the Neulasta injection without incident.

On our deck we have two chair-swings, one has three seats in a row and the other has two seats with a little drink caddy and armrest between them. It was a beautiful evening so I helped her get comfy on the 3-seater and she went to sleep about 5:30. I went out there to check on her every hour or so, but by 11:30 I was ready for bed. I knew she was safe and comfortable on the swing, so I just left her there.

The next morning, Sunday, she slept until 8:30, a total of 15 hours, and she was still pretty groggy. I found it most amusing that not only didn't Chris remember what movie we had seen, but she barely remembered even going! She had no memory of going to the car to get a sucker, and she only faintly recalled her crown popping off. I'm talking "s l e e p y" here, folks!

Kate called, wanting to see how Chris was feeling, and I told her about all the sleeping. Kate's husband, Alan, who is a pharmacist, asked what I had given her and when I told him that she had taken Compazine *and* Ativan, he said, "No wonder she's so sleepy! Either of those alone would have knocked her out!" When she was due for more pills, I gave her the Compazine only and she wasn't quite so tired after that. Or nauseous either; I guess she didn't need both of them. Well, excuuuuuuse me!

I had called our dentist, Dr. Bialecki, who is a personal friend (remember, it's a small town) the previous night to see about getting her crown re-cemented, but she was zonked all evening so I told him I would call the next day and we would figure out when we could coordinate his schedule and her sleeping schedule and make it happen. After several calls, we decided on 9:00 that night!

We went in there and he quickly re-cemented Chris's crown and also made some fluoride trays for her to use during chemo because he said that the drugs are hard on the teeth.

As the days passed, Chris got stronger and stronger and within a short time she was pretty much back to normal. One day, in a casual conversation, Kate happened to mention that she, herself, had never had a surprise party; she had been to many, but none had ever been thrown for her.

That's all that Chris needed, and the planning began. Kate's birthday was coming up the first week of August, but Chris wanted to have the party before her hair started falling out, so we set the date for July 20. We worked with Alan on a scheme to keep Kate busy that day while many of her friends came over to set up our house for the party.

They all arrived around 5:00 bringing food and drinks, with the big surprise scheduled for 5:30. Alan and Kate didn't get to the house until about 6:00, but Kate had had no idea whatsoever and the surprise was complete. Kate was frozen with amazement and kept saying, "What the ---!" over and over again through streaming tears until she got her bearings. Chris had done all of the planning, even though she was going through what she was going through, and Kate and her friends gave her all of the credit that she deserved. Chris had wanted to do something really special for Kate, who had done so much to help us through the cancer process. It was a great success.

Two weeks after her first treatment, Chris found some hair on the pillow; it was falling out right on schedule. Now the serious stuff was going to begin. Forget the two surgeries and the fact that she had a disease that could kill her; *her hair was starting to fall out!* As with everything else, she seemed to take it in stride and we decided to have as much fun with it as we could.

I suggested that as her hair fell out we could use it to make a pillow. She didn't like that idea.

So, we went shopping for a "cranial prosthesis" (I just love that term). We had heard good things about a wig shop at a nearby mall, so we went in. All the choices were fascinating, and "Clarice" was showing Chris some of the various styles. In the process, she mentioned the options for replacing her eyebrows when *they* fell out.

I asked, "Do you have anything to replace her mustache when *it* falls out?" (Chris did not then, nor never has had a mustache.)

I thought I was being pretty funny, and Chris and two nearby customers laughed out loud, but Clarice, with a snap of her fingers and wave of her hand, said, "Honey, step over to the counter and let me show you something."

The "counter" was like a hair toy store, with eyebrows, mustaches, sideburns; you name it. I almost asked about replacement hair for, uh, unmentionable areas but lost my nerve. I think I was more afraid that they *would* have such things than not! I thanked Clarice for the tour and quickly made my way back to the safety of Chris and her wigs.

Chris selected one and we promptly named it "Clarice" for obvious reasons. She also bought a complete eyebrow replacement kit and a few cute hats.

More and more hair started appearing around the house in places where it didn't belong, such as in the sink and on the floor. Before long her head was rag-tag and uneven. Dr. Chap had told us that, when the time came, it would be much more comfortable to just cut it down to about ¼ inch or so and then let *those* fall out naturally.

It was time to see Dale, our favorite stylist at our favorite salon. He has been cutting Chris's and my hair for several years, and is also a personal friend. He has had many clients go through chemotherapy over the years and he knew just what to do. We had decided to have as much fun as we could with it, so he began by cutting off most of the hair on the sides, but leaving the center fairly long. He then moussed it up and formed it into spikes, completing the "Mohawk" look.

I took some photos. Then he taped a safety pin to her eyebrow for the "punk" look. More photos. And finally all she had left was a little peach fuzz.

Then it was my turn. Yes, I was going to cut off my hair since Chris was losing hers, and I must say that it was mildly frightening!

He did pretty much the same with me, styling Mohawk and punk looks with Chris taking the photos. When it was all over, we were the "happy hairless" couple. In fact, I soon began to tell our friends that Chris, with her partly Irish heritage and incredible love for dogs had, in fact, created a whole new breed and that I had the only one: the "Irish Hairless!" (Yes, she *did* think it was funny!)

I was absolutely blown away by how drop-dead cute Chris looked with so little hair. Her head is a wonderful shape and that, coupled with her incredible eyes and beautiful smile made the loss of hair more of a statement than a tragedy. I was also amazed at how much cooler my head felt with so little hair, and when I ran my hand over my new "G.I." cut, I was reminded of how my head felt when I was six years old.

August 1:
2nd Chemotherapy Treatment

I had remembered to order the prescriptions that Chris needed, and she began her Dexamethasone (the steroid) the day before the treatment. I also had ordered the antibiotic, and made an appointment at the local lab for the blood test that she needed to take the day before.

Everything was in order, the blood work was okay, Kate was all set to take care of the animals, and off we went for chemo number two.

I drove, Chris slept, carpool lane… the usual drill.

Georgia was there when we arrived and we all assumed our positions and had a grand old time, talking, laughing, and eating while the poison was going into Chris's arm. This time, though, instead of sandwiches I ordered Thai food, which they actually delivered to us! It seemed sort of like a scene from a movie called "Fast Times at Ridgemont High" where one of the teenage characters (Sean Penn) had a pizza delivered to his history class; it seemed so out of place to have food delivered during chemotherapy!

Dr. Chap came to see Chris (as she did at every treatment) and was very interested to learn how well Chris had tolerated her first treatment. After hearing about how quickly she had bounced back, the surprise party, and how well she had handled the hair loss the doctor proclaimed Chris to be her "poster child" for chemotherapy!

After the treatment, the three of us drove about a block to a small shopping center where Georgia treated us to ice cream at Baskin Robbins. We went to some of the stores in the center, stopping at a bakery and getting some goodies for later, and then walked around the block for the exercise. Everything seemed so normal.

The next day was Friday and Chris was busy working hard around the house doing what she normally does; there seemed to be zero effect from the chemo treatment. I gave her the Neulasta injection, again without incident, and all was well.

Saturday she started feeling pretty punk so we cancelled a dinner date with Gail and Sonia, and Chris spent some time in bed trying to get the room to stop spinning. She didn't want to be as sleepy as she had been for the last treatment, so I only gave her the Compazine and it seemed to do the job.

Sunday Chris was really feeling awful. I planted her in the swing outside and she wanted some fruit, so I returned with an apple and an orange, both cut into sections and arranged in a nice design on the plate. She enjoyed the "presentation" but said she really felt more like watermelon. We happened to have some, so I used her little kitchen tool to make watermelon balls and presented her with a bowl full of them.

She enjoyed that little presentation as well, and began to eat. I left for a few minutes and returned to find that she had vomited on the deck. Perfect! I simply got the hose and washed it off; much easier than if she had vomited in the house! From that point on, she carried a big plastic purple bowl around with her everywhere she went. It turned out to be one of only two times she vomited during her entire course of treatment.

The next day she was hungry, which was always a good sign. Unfortunately she was hungry for something that we didn't have in the house: chili and corn, a concoction that we have enjoyed ever since we were married. It's simple enough: empty a can of corn and a can of chili (we like the chili without beans) into a pot, stir, and heat it up. What could be simpler? It is very tasty and she had a craving for it. We hadn't had it in years, but I went to the market and got several cans of each so we'd have some on hand for later.

> "Sometimes you've just got to do some strange things to keep your patient happy, but I figured that the healing benefits of contentment far outweighed some small inconvenience on my part."

The day after that she had more energy, although not 100 percent. She had a new craving: mashed potatoes, steamed peas, and a Hershey bar with almonds. Hello?? Is she pregnant?? Always aiming to please, I went to a local restaurant and got some mashed potatoes to go, and then to the market to get the peas and Hershey's. Sometimes you've just got to do some strange things to keep your patient happy, but I figured that the healing benefits of contentment far outweighed some small inconvenience on my part.

During this time, as we sat on the swings and enjoyed the deck, I mentioned that we had received a post card from a friend of ours on vacation in Tahiti. It depicted a dreamy lagoon with hotel bungalows stretching out over the water. It looked pretty enticing, especially considering how miserable Chris felt and how stressed and overwhelmed I felt. I suggested that perhaps, when this was all over, we could go there and stay in one of those bungalows.

That started a conversation that lasted for months. I had no idea how I would be able to afford to make such a trip, but the thought of going really gave us energy and put some excitement into some otherwise difficult moments. All we had to do was imagine lying out on the deck of our private overwater bungalow, enjoying the serenity and beauty of Tahiti; it was very energizing. That's when we learned how important it is to have something to look forward to.

By the end of the second week after the treatment most of the little hairs that remained after the "No-Hair Day" had fallen out, and her cute little scalp was populated with a few stray red hairs just above her forehead at the hairline, plus a few randomly placed hairs here and there. She has a perfectly shaped head and I thought she looked adorable. My little cancer patient: I looked at her with mixed feelings of love and disbelief. The love came naturally because she was so physically appealing, because she was so brave about it all, and, well, because I loved her! The disbelief was because I just couldn't believe that this was actually happening to her and, by association, me.

As if Chris didn't have enough to deal with, her postmenopausal hot flashes were continuing. Now that her hair had fallen out, she was a little more comfortable (or should I say less *un*comfortable) when a hot flash occurred because a wet paper towel on her head helped considerably. It used to make me laugh when she would walk around balancing a damp sheet of Job Squad on her head. Kim, Chris's manicurist, used to say that Chris was having "her own personal summer." The hot flashes continued throughout the remainder of her treatment.

The Saturday before her next treatment Georgia drove up to the house and John, Chris's brother, flew down from his home about 30 miles east of San Francisco. John hadn't seen her since all of this began and this was his first opportunity. Besides, Kate had been planning a hat party for Chris that weekend in honor of Chris's hair loss and John and Georgia both wanted to be part of it.

The first thing John did when he got to the house was to produce "Boo-Boo Kitty," a stuffed animal that Chris had given him a couple of years earlier when he was in the hospital after suddenly blacking-out while driving on the freeway. He said, "I thought that Boo-Boo should be with the member of the family that needed her the most." It was very touching.

"That's when we learned how important it is to have something to look forward to."

The first order of business when they arrived was to go for a hike in the forest. The three of them were gone for several hours and had a grand time, as they all love nature and the outdoors. About an hour after they returned, Chris began to feel "itchy" on her left breast and back, and she thought she had brushed up against some poison oak while they were out there. Great. She needs something else to deal with.

We all had a great time together, complete with some dark humor. Chris said, "My brother and sister are both older than I am; they're supposed to die first!" Everyone groaned, and then Chris said to John, "Georgia is going to outlive both of us," referring to some of John's recent medical problems. Georgia, the oldest of the three of them, just laughed.

John piped in, "She already has!" More laughter.

Then Georgia proposed a toast… to me! She thanked me for being so strong and for taking such wonderful care of her baby sister; there wasn't a dry eye in the house. It was very sweet of her and I appreciated it very much.

We told John and Georgia about maybe going to Tahiti. They thought it was a great idea, and we showed them some photos and other information I had found on the Internet. Naturally, they wanted to come along! The more we talked about it, the more excited we got and the more I wondered how I would pay for it.

Sunday was the hat party, held at Kate's house. About 30 of Kate's and Chris's friends showed up, each wearing a hat and bringing one for Chris. There was a ton of food brought in "pot luck" style by the closest friends, and everyone had a grand time watching Chris open all of her gifts, which were in every color and style imaginable. Some were heavy and warm for winter; others were light and airy for summer. Each had its own "personality" and it was truly heartwarming that so many people did so much for Chris. Kate really went all out and it was a smashing success.

The last hat to be opened was in a very large box, and was from Dale, our hair stylist, and his companion Glenn.

When Chris removed the colorful wrapping, there was an office-style storage box, and when she opened it and saw what was inside she laughed out loud. She reached into the box and removed a Carmen Miranda-style hat, about 12 inches high, covered with artificial fruit. (I invite you to visit **www.CancerForTwo.com/c42book** to see a short video clip of this event – you'll love it!) Dale and Glenn had constructed the hat using an adjustable baseball cap as a base, so Chris and Glenn fiddled with it until it fit just right, and she put it on to everyone's delight. "It was fabulous!" This hat would prove to be a source of great fun as the treatments wore on and on.

That night, I flew up to the San Francisco area with John as I had a conference to attend in San Francisco. I stayed with John and Patty, his wonderful significant-other whom we all adore, and used his pickup truck to drive back and forth to BART, the train that took me to and from the city. On Tuesday night I was on the road to see an old friend when Chris called me on the cell phone.

"I don't think my poison oak is poison oak after all. I just figured out what it probably really is," she told me with a dreadful tone in her voice.

"Tell me."

"Shingles."

My heart sank like a stone. Shingles is an after-effect of chicken pox, a common childhood disease. The chicken pox virus hides in the spinal column and, if it comes out at all, strikes at times of great stress or weakness. It follows the nerves from its hiding place in the spine and takes the form of extremely painful sores and lesions, usually in a pattern on the torso from the chest, across one side of the body and around to the spine. I had known only a couple of people who had had Shingles and they were extremely uncomfortable for six to ten weeks. *WEEKS!*

"It's got to be. I knew I didn't see any poison oak on our hike, my immune system is compromised because of the chemotherapy, and I've had chicken pox. It's exactly the way I've heard it described; it itches like crazy and the red spots and scabs are spreading in that pattern."

We discussed it a little more and she said she would call Dr. Win first thing in the morning to see if there was anything that could be done.

I felt badly for her. How much more does this poor woman have to take? I felt terrible that I wasn't there with her, but when this trip was planned we both thought that it would come at the best possible time: the last few days before a chemo treatment (the next one was the day after I returned) and, therefore, the maximum number of days since the previous treatment when she would be feeling her best.

The next day Dr. Win did, indeed, confirm Chris's self-diagnosis and gave her some anti-viral drugs, but there was bad news: those drugs usually don't help much unless they are taken within 48 to 72 hours of the first appearance of symptoms. The itching started Saturday but she didn't get the prescription until Wednesday, which meant that she was about 24 hours too late. She was in for a rough ride.

August 23:
3rd Chemotherapy Treatment

Two hour drive, Chris sleeping, carpool lane, watch for red lights…

Georgia had once again taken the afternoon off to be with us. It was pretty much the same as it always was, although this time I went to get the Thai food, which was just across the street.

This chemo we spent a lot of time talking about Chris's new problem: Shingles. The nurses and Dr. Chap concurred with our notion that the chemotherapy put enough stress on Chris's immune system to reactivate the chicken pox virus that lay dormant in her nervous system. I started making calls on the cell phone, beginning with our dermatologist and also the dermatologist of a friend, trying to get some sort of relief for the itching and pain that Chris was suffering. After a number of calls and callbacks, I finally got the name of a cream that contained cortisone, which acted like a local anesthetic: Ela-Max. It used to be prescription-only but had just become over-the-counter. The nurse that recommended it warned me, though, that it was expensive.

There was a pharmacy in the building, so I went over there to see if he had Ela-Max cream and, sure enough, he did! I was thrilled. A 30-ounce tube (like a tube of toothpaste) was $75; I wasn't so thrilled. That seemed outrageous to me, so I walked three blocks to a major drug store chain to see what their price was for comparison: $94 for the same thing, and they would have to order it; would I like to come in the next day? Sure, I'm going to drive two hours each way to spend even more money on this than I had to!

I went back to the first pharmacy, took a deep breath, and forked over the $75. I thought it was pretty ironic that the only cream I was able to get was non-prescription, and therefore not covered by insurance. Oh, what the heck: I'll just pick a few twenty dollar bills off of the money tree that's growing in our yard and that will cover it. If it helps her, of course the money doesn't matter, but still…

We had arrived a little late for this treatment and there had been some delays, so Chris wasn't finished until about 6:15 p.m. when we discovered, much to our delight, that the attendant in the parking booth had left for the evening and we didn't have to pay for parking! We followed Georgia over to one of her favorite Italian restaurants and had a charming meal in a lovely setting.

That night I had a dream about Chris. In the dream, there was a leopard just off of our deck and a dog that was in trouble. Chris, ever the dog lover even in my dreams, went down to save the dog and at one point had the leopard draped around her neck and was twirling it around and around. In the dream, I went to get my video camera and was frustrated over and over again trying to get there to tape the action. My interpretation of that dream was that I was very impressed with Chris and how brave she was to face this with such courage, and how frustrated I was that I couldn't do anything to help.

This treatment had been on a Friday, and Saturday Chris felt pretty good. Her shingles were really starting to become painful, though, and even the rubbing of a light T-shirt was extremely uncomfortable for her, so I came up with an idea: let's take an old T-shirt and cut out the area that would be touching the shingles lesions. We found a very old shirt of mine and I got the scissors. She put it on and I cut out the area v e r y c a r e f u l l y a n d s l o w l y. Unfortunately, I didn't do it carefully or slowly enough, because I touched the extremely sensitive area with the tip of the scissors. YIKES! It gives me the creeps just writing about it! She yelped and yanked the scissors away from me and that was the end of my career as a clothing designer.

Later that day I went to retrieve the Neulasta injection from the refrigerator and discovered, to my horror, that Chris had accidentally put it in the freezer instead of the refrigerator when we returned home the previous evening. We always brought a cooler on our long drives in order to have fresh, cold bottles of water when we needed them. When we left each treatment, they gave us the Neulasta injection in a zip-lock bag with a block of frozen gel to keep it cool until we got home. We always put the zip-lock in the cooler for the ride home, and then Chris, being the efficient person she is, put everything away before we went to bed. She saw the frozen gel in the bag but not the Neulasta, so she put the bag in the freezer. Oops.

I wasn't sure what to do, how best to thaw it, or even if it was usable. And it was Saturday. I tend to be fairly positive about things like this so I called Amgen, the manufacturer, and thought (hoped) maybe someone would be there, even on the weekend. My philosophy about such things is that "it's better to call and be wrong than *not* to call and be wrong." If no one was there, I could try a pharmacy.

Whaddaya know: there was someone at Amgen! And, it was someone who knew her stuff; she said that I should place it in the refrigerator for about an hour to thaw, then leave it at room temperature for about 30 minutes before administering the injection. It would be okay to use as long as it wasn't frozen a second time, in which case it would have to be discarded. I followed her instructions and everything turned out fine.

The next evening, Sunday, Chris started to feel the effects of the chemo and Monday morning she was feeling pretty nauseated. I heard what I thought was the sound of vomiting, so I ran toward the sound and found Chris hunched over the bathroom sink. I didn't know whether to help or go away, and I was horrified to see her like that.

After it was over, I asked her what she would have preferred, so I'd know what to do if it happened again. Should I hold her forehead like my mother used to do for me when I was sick as a child, or should I go away and give her some privacy? She told me to hang around in case she needed me, but not to touch her. Fair enough. Hopefully we wouldn't need to use this little bit of information. We didn't: that was the last time that she got that sick.

Part of the reason that Chris got as sick as she did was that she didn't want to take the anti-nausea medications unless she needed them; she didn't like the way they made her so sleepy. After this incident she agreed that she should take something on the evening of the second day after the treatments whether she thought she needed it or not. Dr. Chap had given us three anti-nausea drugs; Compazine and Ativan, which we had been using, and Zofran which we had not. Dr. Chap had told us that the Zofran was about $30 a pill so we didn't even fill the prescription until we found out if the others would be sufficient. We did, however, have some samples.

Chris took one and the nausea went away almost immediately, and stayed away; plus, it didn't make her the least bit sleepy. Perfect: that's why they were *worth* $30 a pill! We decided to fill that prescription after all; to my relief, insurance paid the bulk of it.

While all of this was going on, the shingles were getting worse. The lesions were blistering and breaking and the entire area looked pretty nasty. I could only imagine how uncomfortable it was. So, in addition to the antibiotics and Zofran she was taking, we threw some pain pills into the mix. It turned out that the Ela-Max *did* help her and we used it sparingly, but it soon became evident that one tube wasn't going to do the job. Kate called around and found that Costco's pharmacy had the best price (no surprise, really), $42, but it would take 24 hours to get it. No problem there, since we would have plenty of advance notice of running out, so we ordered two more tubes.

Several times a day I was called upon to apply the Ela-Max to the affected area. To get an idea of the size of that area, imagine placing the palm of your hand over the middle of your chest, and then moving your hand to the left, under your arm, and then over your back to your spine. Almost all of the skin that would have fallen under the palm of your hand during that motion was affected. It was rough and full of blisters, scabs, and caked blood. I covered the area with the Ela-Max using the tip of my index finger to spread the cream very carefully and slowly, so as not to hurt her even more. I felt so sorry for her having to deal with all of this at the same time; tears filled my eyes as I spread the cream. She was so brave, hardly ever complained, continued to do as much as she could around the house, and still had a pleasant attitude most of the time in spite of the pain.

I continued to do most of the "heavy lifting" around the house, taking care of plants and animals alike, and still fretting over our money situation and trying to get some work done. Even when I did do the work, I wasn't bringing in much money and if it weren't for the residual income from my software I honestly don't know what we would have done. It was becoming evident that my business as "The Stay-at-Home CEO" was not happening. I was using a consultant who had warned me what a tough market I was in: there were a lot of dreamers and people who wanted to make lots of money with no work, wouldn't (or couldn't) spend anything to learn how, and there were a lot of "gurus" out there offering up the same sort of advice that I was. What the heck was I going to do?

On top of that, I was so consumed with our own situation that I missed a friend's birthday as well as following-up on several other friends' illnesses and issues. I felt like I was being a bad friend and, even though I had a good reason to be distracted and everyone understood, it made me feel even worse. It hadn't been the first time during Chris's illness that this had happened, and it wouldn't be the last.

> "... it is absolutely essential that the caregiver take some time for him/herself. As the flight attendant says in the pre-flight instructions, 'Put on your own oxygen mask before helping others with theirs.'"

My mood cycles continued; happy, sad, stressed, afraid, overwhelmed, and back to happy again. They finally took their toll on me about a week after the third chemo treatment and I began to get a taste of Chris's discomfort when a small lesion appeared on my stomach, just above my belly button. Oh... my... God..." I thought. "I'm getting shingles too!" Fear settled over me like a blanket and I realized just how brave Chris really was. I told her, "If this is really shingles, I don't know if I can be as brave as you are."

I remembered the 72-hour rule and went to see Dr. Win immediately. She took a look and said that she wasn't going to call it shingles, even though it *looked* like shingles, because there was only a single lesion. Shingles, she told me, usually took a pattern that wrapped the torso from the middle of the front to the middle of the back, like Chris's case. She did, however, give me Valtrex, the anti-viral medication, just in case.

The one sore, about the size of a dime, was painful and annoying and I couldn't help but think of Chris and her affected area, which was the size of several dollar bills. How could she stand this? My "sympathy shingle" went away in about 2 weeks and I'll never know if the Valtrex saved me or not, but I felt that I got off pretty easily.

Another big issue was coming to a head during this time: there would be a total eclipse of the sun in December off the southern coast of Africa. Naturally, I wanted to go because, as I said earlier, I intend to go to every total eclipse for the rest of my life. But more than that I *needed* to go because I had been under heavy stress for quite a while and, frankly, I needed the break. I felt guilty then for feeling that way, and I feel guilty about it right now as I'm writing this, but the truth of the matter is that it is absolutely essential that the caregiver take some time for him/herself. As the flight attendant says in the pre-flight instructions, "Put on your own oxygen mask before helping others with theirs."

Another reason to plan this trip was the importance of having something to look forward to. We both knew how energizing our talk about Tahiti was, and I knew that this would do the same for me. I was quite excited about the possibilities of going to see another eclipse and the thought of it brightened my darker moments.

There were, however, a number of complications and considerations.

The first one, as I'm sure you can imagine, was the money. Africa is never an inexpensive proposition although this trip would not be as expensive as most because I was able to get a substantial discount on an eclipse cruise as well as the airfare. All of my recent eclipse adventures had been financed with money that I inherited from my mother when she died in 1999. I had put it aside in a special "eclipse" account and used it only for eclipse travel, which I know would have made her happy. I considered that money to be sacred; if I had to dip into it for day-to-day expenses, that would indicate that we were at the beginning of the end of our resources, and it had been about just that possibility that I had been so worried over the preceding months.

The bigger issue, however, was whether I could leave Chris for the amount of time I would have to be gone. That depended on the timing of her treatments; at this point in her treatment plan it looked like the last chemo treatment would be on October 24 and, with an ideal break of three to six weeks, radiation should start no later than December 5. The eclipse was December 4. If I was going to go to the eclipse, clearly Chris would have to go to her first few radiation treatments without me and she had no problem with that whatsoever. We knew that the first two or three weeks of radiation were going to be a breeze, so that wasn't a concern.

On the other hand, if some complication should arise between now and then I would cancel the trip in a heartbeat in order to stay home with her. That meant that cancellation provisions would be crucial to any trip that I planned.

The final consideration was that space was filling up (believe it or not there are lots of eclipse chasers out there who clamor for available space on eclipse expeditions) and my special discount was only available if I booked the trip by the end of August.

Chris as well as all of our friends and relatives were encouraging me to go. I was the only one who had any hesitation whatsoever, and that was due to my perhaps exaggerated sense of responsibility for everything that happened to Chris, but Chris said that she would be fine, and if anything came up she had Kate and other friends nearby who would jump in to help. In fact, Chris knew how important eclipses are to me and said that *she* would feel guilty if I *didn't* go because of her. It's not as if I could simply delay the trip until treatment was over; eclipses only happen when they happen and there will only be a limited number of them during my lifetime.

I decided that I would rather book the trip and be wrong than not book the trip and be wrong. If I had to forfeit some of the money because Chris had a complication, so be it. I wasn't going to give up any possibility of going because something *might* happen that would prevent it. Besides, the value of having that to look forward to would make the risk worthwhile.

I booked the trip on August 30; I would leave at midnight of Thanksgiving Day and return on December 10. The anticipation began to work its magic and almost immediately I had renewed energy and optimism.

> **"The anticipation began to work its magic and almost immediately I had renewed energy and optimism."**

On the morning of September 11 I was working early when Chris, who is usually not up at that hour even when she is feeling well, called me in the office and said that I should come upstairs to see what they were doing at the school. The northern boundary of our property is the southern boundary of an elementary school, but we don't really see or hear them much because that boundary is also the crest of a hill, which is high enough to block the view and sound. If we walk to the top of our property, though, we can see the parking lot and part of the playground as well as a spectacular vista of the surrounding mountains and desert beyond. Chris had been up there in her robe, enjoying the scenery on a beautiful, balmy morning when the ceremony at the school had begun.

When I got there the kids were all sitting on the ground and there were some government officials there, as well as a sheriff and fireman. The children all sang God Bless America and it was very touching. Standing there among the beautiful pines and looking out over the majestic mountains, hearing a gentle breeze rustling the leaves and pine needles, it was unimaginable that the evil that perpetrated the events of September 11 could exist in the world. I wondered what kind of world those kids would live to see, and I understood the fear and uncertainty that my parents must have gone through during World War II. Sure, the generation after that war studied it but we knew how it all ended. Now I knew how it felt to wonder how it would end and what would happen next, just as our parents must have done.

Surrounded by all of this beauty, and seeing Chris with her perfectly shaped but almost-bald head and realizing our own personal challenges, plus the touching reminder of such an awful day, I began quaking with emotion and couldn't hold back the tears. Later that day I called the principal of the school, told her that I was their neighbor and had "eavesdropped" on their ceremony, and that I thought it was a wonderful tribute and so appropriate for the children.

There was little else on the news besides the September 11 anniversary; stories, photos, and video from that awful day. Chris and I were talking about how difficult it was to watch and she said that when she saw the women who had lost their husbands, had to raise children on their own, are financially strapped, and were losing their homes, she realized that what she was going through was a "walk in the park." I guess it's all in your perspective, isn't it?

She told me that she had learned that point of view from my mother, who had watched her brother battle polio in the 1950's. He was in an iron lung for six months, and was left severely handicapped for the rest of his life. Shortly afterwards his wife died of cancer and he had to raise three small children; through it all he was one of the nicest and funniest people I've ever known. Mom always said that whenever she thought she had problems, she just looked at him and his wonderful attitude and realized she didn't have anything to complain about. As I write this I can feel her smiling down from above at this wonderful, positive influence she had on both Chris and me and now, hopefully, on you as well.

Tomorrow was the next chemo appointment so Chris had to have her blood test at the local hospital. While she was

---

"Chris . . . said that when she saw the women who had lost their husbands, had to raise children on their own, are financially strapped, and were losing their homes, she realized that what she was going through was a 'walk in the park.'"

---

gone, I realized that we were almost out of Ela-Max and, since our nearest Costco was in the city and 45 minutes away, it would be very convenient to pick up more while we were down there the next day. The problem was that we would be going by there at 11:30 a.m. and 9:00 p.m., but the pharmacy delivery was at 2:00 p.m. and they closed at 8:30. That meant that we couldn't get it there, so I found another Costco that wasn't too far from the chemo treatment office and ordered it from *that* pharmacy. We would pick it up after the treatment but before dinner. Two more tubes, thankyou-verymuch.

September 12:
4ᵗʰ Chemotherapy Treatment

We got to chemo about 10 minutes late but it wasn't a problem. It was pretty much like the other treatments; Georgia was there and I went across the street to get Thai food for lunch. There was a slight difference, however: Chris wore her "Carmen Miranda" hat, which was a big hit with everyone in the office: staff and patients alike. How could you not smile when you see that hat? How could you not wonder how she had the nerve to wear it?

Dr. Chap was blown away when she saw Chris's head piled high with plastic fruit, and just couldn't believe that Chris would wear it in public.

We were ready to leave about 15 minutes before the parking attendant left for the day, so we waited! After he left, we did too and Georgia followed us to Costco so we could pick up the Ela-Max. Believe it or not, Chris wore that hat into the store, walking around like there was nothing out of the ordinary. Heads were turning everywhere; it was quite a sight. I was so glad I brought my camera; you can see a photo at **www.CancerForTwo.com/c42book** .

After that, Georgia led us on a surface-street "tour" of Los Angeles, trying to find a particular Chinese restaurant. It turned out to be much farther than she thought it would be and we didn't start eating until after 8:00! By the time we got home it was almost 11:00 p.m. and Chris was sound asleep in the back of the 4Runner. I didn't want to bother her, so I did my evening chores, walking dogs and feeding horses; I finally got to bed at 12:15 and Chris was still asleep in the car, so I left her there. Why disturb her when she was so comfortable? When she was ready she would get up and make her way to the bedroom.

That weekend there was a 3-day conference in Palm Springs held by my local chapter of the National Speakers Association. I wanted to attend but it was out of the question because I knew that Chris would come crashing down on Saturday or Sunday and I needed to be there. I did, however, want to at least go to the opening session on Friday night (the night after her treatment) and, since it was only about 90 minutes away, I figured I could do that and come back that same night. The day after the treatment is usually pretty normal, so I planned on doing that with the option of canceling at the last minute if Chris needed me to be there. I felt guilty as hell for leaving her, but she seemed to be doing all right. She said, "You have to have your own life! I'm fine; go ahead and go. If I have a problem I'll call you on the cell phone."

I got about 3 miles away and realized I hadn't given her the Neulasta injection, so I had to come back home. It wasn't frozen this time (!) so it went smoothly and I only ended up being about 30 minutes late to the conference.

I got home late, so by the time I cut up the carrots and took them to the horses, walked the dogs, cleaned the cat boxes, and cleaned and covered Poncho, it was 1:15 a.m. when I finally fell into bed.

The next morning Chris and I both slept in, finally getting out of bed around 9:30. She was feeling pretty groggy and took a Zofran to head off the nausea that was sure to come. It seemed to work, because she never did get sick.

I made her some oatmeal and tended to the dogs, cats, parrot, and horses. By the time I was finished and fed myself, it was almost time for lunch!! It was a beautiful day, so Chris and I sat out on the swings and just sort of existed together, making small talk and enjoying the weather and each other. It all seemed so sweet and normal, except for the big purple bowl she had with her, just in case.

The fatiguing effect of the treatments was cumulative, which means that the effects of each treatment were a little worse than the previous ones. It is the whole idea of chemotherapy to not let the body completely recover from one treatment before administering another because if the body could recover, so could the cancer cells that we were trying to kill.

At that point I remembered that the Alpenhorn News, the local paper for which I wrote a weekly column, was having an open house to show off their new offices. I wanted to go but didn't want to leave Chris. She told me that she was probably going to sleep all day anyway so I should go ahead, which I did. When I got back she was just getting up and was hungry so I heated up some of the chicken pie that Anne and Terry had brought us from a restaurant in the city a few days earlier (Chris was only eating it a little at a time). Then I made a tuna and noodle casserole using a recipe my sister had given me that my mother had used when I was little, bringing back all sorts of childhood memories.

Although I had already known this, it struck me as I was making that dinner that it was very smart to make large meals, then refrigerate or freeze the leftovers. It may not appeal to everyone's palate, but in these circumstances efficiency is probably more important than fancy meals and it makes sense to maximize the output from the time you spend cooking. From that point on I made casseroles or double recipes for that very reason; it took virtually the same amount of my time to prepare a recipe versus a double portion of that same recipe, so it was like cooking two or three meals all at once! A great way to save time and still provide the food.

Another big time saver is the crock-pot. Throw a few things in and let it cook all day, the crock-pot is another way to prepare multiple meals in a short amount of time.

"... minimize the effort and maximize the output when it comes to making meals."

My advice is to minimize the effort and maximize the output when it comes to making meals. Even if you decide to order take out or have something delivered, get enough for more than one meal; bring home eight tacos instead of four, order an extra large pizza instead of the large, etc.

Anyway, as I prepared the tuna and noodles, I put Planes, Trains, and Automobiles in the VCR, which is one of our favorite movies of all time, and that always puts a smile on my face. Then it was time to walk and feed the dogs, feed the horses, do the dishes, etc. Will this ever end? I was getting so discouraged.

When Chris went back to bed I went in there to "tuck her in" and make sure that she had everything she needed, that the walkie-talkie radio was set to the correct channel, etc. She took my hand and gave me a look I'll never forget.

"Thank you for taking such good care of me. I don't know what I would have done without you."

Suddenly, it was all worthwhile. I told her, "Thank *you* for being a good and brave patient. You make it easy."

It is important to express your appreciation to your patient and to those who help you, and to do it with heartfelt sincerity. The positive impact of a kind word cannot be overstated, and that goes for the patient as well as the caregiver.

The next day she was feeling pretty awful; not so much nauseated, but just a general weakness and malaise. It was another beautiful day so I parked her on one of the deck swings and got some food (and the big purple bowl). There wasn't much else I could do except simply "be" with her, so that's what I did.

A week after the treatment she was beginning to get her energy back and the weather wasn't too hot, so we thought we could make our annual pilgrimage to the Los Angeles

County Fair. This is a major annual event for us and we hadn't missed one since we met in 1978.

As I have mentioned, we are normally fairly health conscious and eat accordingly, although we are not fanatics about it. Perhaps "aware" would be a better word to describe our health-related eating habits. The Fair, however, is loaded with the most outrageous and unhealthy food you can imagine, so we have decreed it to be our "one-day-of-the-year-anything-goes-no-holds-barred-junk-food-pigout" and we eat whatever looks good no matter what. Variety, not quantity, is the order of the day, and we split just about everything we get so we don't fill up on any one thing. Sometimes, just for fun, we keep track of all of the different foods that we've eaten during our day at the fair, and it's always quite a list. For example, one day's "take" might include four lemonades, hot dog on a stick, egg roll, cinnamon roll, Kettle Corn, chocolate milk, French dip sandwich, onion rings, two tacos, butter toffee peanuts, apple crisps, funnel cake, another hot dog on a stick, another cinnamon roll, ice cream dots, churro, Italian Sausage on a stick, cheese cake dipped in chocolate on a stick (I'm not kidding), and so on. Oh, and the exhibits are interesting too!

There was no way we were going to miss the Fair that year, so we picked a day between chemo treatments when it wasn't too hot (it can get pretty miserable at the Fair) and went for it. We rented an electric cart for Chris so she wouldn't waste her limited energy walking everywhere (and there is a considerable amount of walking... one year I brought a pedometer and measured over 7 miles that day). The cart did the trick and she was fine the entire day. We had a grand time and, for that day anyway, we forgot about cancer and chemotherapy and insufficient income and no time or

"The importance of a kind word cannot be overstated."

inclination to work and overwhelm and stress and doctors and appointments, etc.

It was only a few days after that that I was supposed to start on blood pressure medication. For the previous six months or so my blood pressure had been creeping up, and I had asked nurses at Chris's various appointments to take my blood pressure in order to keep an eye on it. Dr. Win was not happy with the readings and, although it was not really "high" in the classic sense, it was just on the cusp and she wanted to get it under control, especially considering the stress of our situation.

I felt distinctly uneasy about taking the medication. For one thing, it felt like a sign of old age that I was beginning my first medication for a chronic condition. Geez! I remember my mother taking a slew of pills every day for various ailments and wondered if this was the beginning for me. The other thing that made me uneasy, and I'm ashamed to admit it, was that it was a new medication and I didn't know how it might affect me. When I identified this fear I had a good laugh at myself; my poor wife is taking about 5 different medications, chemotherapy, surgeries, etc., and I'm worried about a blood pressure pill?? What a baby! I said to myself, "Take it and shut the hell up!" So I did, and my blood pressure improved with no side effects.

Life continued as it always did between chemo treatments. Chris gradually got more and more energy and did more and more of her normal chores around the house, pushing her personal envelope because she doesn't like to sit or lie around doing nothing. And, as she did more and more, I tended to take it as a personal affront because I felt like she was doing more than she really should because she didn't feel confident that I could do it "properly." If I mentioned that to her she would roll her eyes at me and tell me not to be ridiculous, and then I would be okay with it. Until the next time. Color me overly sensitive and protective.

> # "It was a good reminder for her that life *does* get back to normal and that this ordeal *will* end."

About two weeks into this treatment cycle, Chris treated herself to a pedicure. Also, Dennis, Kathy's husband, came over so we could meet their new dog, and he told us about a momma bear and her two cubs that were going through the dumpster at the school. In fact, he told us, the lid on one of the dumpsters had fallen closed, trapping one of the cubs inside and they had to rescue the little guy the next morning. Momma bear had beaten the heck out of the dumpster lid trying to get it open.

That night, Chris treated me to dinner because I was such a good caregiver (there's that appreciation thing again), and, on the way home we decided to drive by the dumpsters at the school to see the damage. When we got there, we couldn't believe our luck: all three of the bears were there! As soon as we drove up, the momma bear stood upright on her hind legs to appear as large as possible, and the babies scampered up a nearby tree. After a while, the cubs came slowly down and the three of them lumbered off together.

The next day, Chris felt well enough to go riding on her beloved Keno, and I went along on Kelly. We spent lots of time with the horses both before and after the ride, and I know it did wonders for Chris's spirits. It was a good reminder for her that life *does* get back to normal and that this ordeal *will* end.

It was about this time that Chris started to notice that she was getting cuts and sores inside and on the corners of her mouth. It was quite painful and she was extremely sensitive to spicy foods, so I hit the Internet and came up with "Mucositis," another common side effect of chemotherapy that we didn't know about. (What *else* don't we know about??) I called Dr. Chap's office and spoke to Joan, who told us about a rinse that can be ordered that usually helps this sort of thing. If that didn't work, there was a preparation called "Gel-Clair" that we could buy.

Joan called in a prescription for the rinse and Chris tried it. Not only did it taste horrible and sting like hell, it didn't help. So then, on the Friday before Labor Day weekend, the search began for Gel-Clair. None of the pharmacies we called had it in stock and all were willing to order it but, because of the long weekend, they wouldn't have it until Tuesday. WRONG! Chris was really uncomfortable and that makes me crazy so there was no way I was going to make her wait four days; Kate helped out by making calls to try to find someone, anyone, that had it in stock so that I could pick it up that day. No one did. She called the distributor; no luck. She even called the manufacturer; they told us to call the distributor. Finally, we found a pharmacy that was open on Saturdays, so they could order it and have it the very next day.

I was itching to go for a motorcycle ride anyway, so the next day I took my bike down to the city to pick it up. Not only did I get the prescription *Chris* desperately needed, but I got to go for a ride which *I* desperately needed.

The Gel-Clair helped, but not much, so now that the shingles were winding down, she had to deal with this intense pain in her mouth. As Anne said, "What's next? Locusts??"

It was about this time that we got some bad news from Kathy, our neighbor. She, her husband Dennis, and we had been working on solving a problem with teenagers that were riding their off-road motorcycles in the forest next to our house. Besides damaging the vegetation and causing ruts that eventually begin to erode, there is a distinct danger of forest fires. The areas in question are either federally or privately owned and motorcycles are expressly forbidden. The motor-cyclists were gaining access to the forest by riding in the narrow corridor between our property and the elementary school, so Dennis arranged for a barrier to be installed that would allow pedestrians into the forest but keep out the motorcycles.

There were other people in the neighborhood, though, that used that same corridor for riding their horses into the forest and they strongly objected to the barrier. Kathy had been talking to one such woman who told her, unaware that Kathy was our neighbor, that "Those Balches [that's us] installed the barrier because they didn't want anyone riding horses in 'their' forest. They don't want anyone back there but themselves."

Spreading false rumors in the neighborhood about Chris is not something you want to do.

When Chris found out she immediately picked up the phone and called the woman and confronted her about it. Not exactly what you would call the confrontational type, I just shook my head in amazement and cowered in the corner.

"I never said that," the woman told her sweetly and innocently. "Why would I go around spreading a rumor like that? I'm not that sort of person."

"Why would someone make that up?" Chris wanted to know. (Who were we going to believe, Kathy or this woman? The answer was pretty obvious. Besides, that woman used to board her horse with a friend of ours down the street, and she was summarily kicked off of their property because she was such a troublemaker.) "I have breast cancer and I'm going through chemotherapy. I don't need more stress caused by lies told about me to the neighbors. The school constructed that barrier, not us, to keep the motorcycles out. We love horses and we would never try to stop you from going back there."

You tell her, Chris! Good for you!

Soon after that we took the 4Runner to a dealer in the city because I felt that the shocks were wearing out. After 150,000 miles, it's probably time to have a look. The dealership called to tell me that the truck did need shocks and a few other things to the tune of almost $1,000. Just what I needed, more money spent. I had recently spent over $600 on that car for a new radiator and tune-up.

That really sent me on a tailspin about work, career, and money. I felt completely lost; what was I going to do to make money? I didn't feel I knew anything that anyone would want to know or learn, or who would hire me as a consultant... consult about what? 8-year-old computer technology?? Hopeless is a good word to describe the feeling. At this point I didn't even feel like doing anything worthwhile... too afraid that I would look like an idiot and everything just seemed like sooooooo much work. When you're on the edge as I was, it doesn't take much to send you into an abyss of despair. Even though I recognized intellectually why I was feeling so down, it didn't seem to help much. A good night's sleep didn't change anything, but it left me better equipped to deal with it.

A Word About Sex During Chemotherapy

H^{a!}

October 3:
5th Chemo Treatment

Kate was working today to take care of the animals. We rode in to town: serenity, Chris sleeping, carpool lane, watching for flashing lights in rearview mirror... it was the usual ride into the city.

We arrived on time (for us) and Iris, another of the chemotherapy nurses, got the IV inserted properly on the first "stick." Georgia arrived and we talked and laughed and ate Thai food again. I even, actually, did some work on my laptop; it was the first time I had done anything on it, even though I had brought it to all of the previous chemotherapy treatments.

Georgia's birthday had been the previous week, so after the treatment we went to our favorite Japanese restaurant, about 20 minutes away, to celebrate. What a great meal we had, laughing and joking the entire time.

The very next day, Chris felt well enough to go for a horseback ride so the two of us went because we both knew she would be feeling terrible for the next week or so. And, that night, Chris treated me to dinner at one of my favorite restaurants. Gail and Sonia met us there and we had a wonderful time with good friends and good food.

The following Thursday night, a week after the treatment, Chris was feeling pretty punk but was able to move around fairly well on her own, so she encouraged me to go to the meeting of the Book Publicists of Southern California, an organization to which I belong. The meeting is about 90 miles away, and required that I be gone from about 4:00 in the afternoon to 11:00 that night. I felt pretty guilty about leaving her but, once again, she told me that I had to have my own life and that she would be okay for a few hours. She was fine while I was gone, although it was a little creepy because my cell phone didn't work due to an electrical problem in the car and I couldn't get hold of her. By the time I got home and did all of the evening chores, it was almost 2:00 a.m.

Needless to say, I slept later the next day but Chris was doing fine after this treatment and was pretty much self-sufficient, even though her mucositis (mouth sores) was really painful. The entire day was filled with chores and interruptions; my frustration level was barely tolerable as I was able to do nothing that seemed like progress.

The next day was going to be a big day, because I went to a chapter meeting for The National Speakers Association followed by dinner with Sean, an old friend from Yosemite National Park whom we hadn't seen for years; he happened to be staying nearby for a seminar, so he called to make arrangements to get together. The chapter meeting was 86 miles away, so I had to get up at 5:15 a.m. in order to do the horse chores before I left. As soon as I got home from the meeting I showered and changed and Sean arrived. We gave him a tour of the house and barn, then went to dinner. Naturally, when we got back I had all of the nightly animal chores to do.

The next day I was extremely tired, and so was Chris. Even though she slept both before and after our visit with Sean, she still didn't have much energy and all that talking wore her out. We had a lazy day on the deck swings, reading and just hanging out together.

I guess that the main thing to emphasize here is that life during chemo isn't as bad as I thought it would be. Sure, I was overloaded with chores and things to do, but I was still able to maintain many of my activities in spite of it all and Chris was, as usual, very brave and strong and did as much as she could as soon as she could.

Now, with the last chemo treatment scheduled and in sight, it was time to begin the extremely complicated scheduling for the 2nd stage reconstruction surgery as well as the startup of radiation. Here were the considerations, some of which I didn't discover until I began working on it:

- Dr. Da Lio wanted to do the reconstruction surgery about three weeks after the last chemo treatment.
- Dr Da Lio had to see Chris prior to scheduling the procedure.
- Chris could not do anything for the first week after the chemo treatment because of fatigue.
- There also had to be a pre-operative appointment with the anesthesiologist.
- Since radiation treatments would be every day, Monday through Friday, for six weeks, it would not be practical to have radiation performed at UCLA because it was just too far away, so we chose Loma Linda University Medical Center, which is only 45 minutes away and has a world-class reputation.
- Radiation had to begin, ideally, no later than six weeks after the last chemo treatment.
- In order to begin radiation therapy, Chris had to undergo a "simulation" where they do precise calculations and measurements. This was to be done at a separate appointment.
- In order to schedule the simulation, she had to have a consult with the radiologist.
- In order to schedule the consult, we had to have Chris's complete medical history, lab tests, etc. copied and sent to the Loma Linda radiologist.
- The radiologist only did consults and simulations on Thursdays.
- Thanksgiving was in the middle of all of this.
- I was leaving for Africa at 11:55 p.m., the night of Thanksgiving.

All of these appointments had to be completed, in proper sequence of course, so that radiation treatments could begin within the preferred time frame. Can you feel the stress? I can feel my chest tightening up just writing the list!

It was obvious to me that the sooner I began working on this the more likely I could pull it off, but Dr. Da Lio's office couldn't schedule anything until we knew when the last chemo treatment was going to be. Now that I had that date, October 24, the phone calls to make all of the appointments began.

I'll spare you the gory details; suffice it to say that everything was scheduled and it all fit together perfectly, even though there was a problem getting all of the medical records copied and sent. It was a lot of work and worry, and I got a tremendous amount of help from UCLA who not only coordinated several appointments, but managed to get several of them scheduled on the same day in order to minimize the number of trips we had to make.

Some of the scheduling had to wait until we saw Dr. Da Lio, which was scheduled for three days before the final chemo treatment when Chris would be feeling her best. That saved us several weeks that would be needed for Chris's recovery from that treatment. We estimated that the surgery would be the second week of November so we scheduled the radiation consult and simulation for the week after that. Radiation would begin December 3rd and, although I would be in Africa at that time, neither of us were worried about it because we had been told that the beginning of the radiation is a breeze; it was the last treatments that can be difficult. However, nothing was going to stop me from feeling guilty about being gone even though it was more of an emotional issue than a practical one.

By the time that the last chemo treatment rolled around, everything was set for the next six weeks and I didn't have to worry about it.

Much.

October 21:
Another Surgical Consult

The Monday before the Thursday of the last chemo treatment we went to see Dr. Da Lio in order to determine the best course of action for the 2nd stage reconstruction surgery. It was the usual "UCLA day" routine: Kate worked so she could take care of the animals, I drove in and enjoyed the serenity, Chris slept, and we didn't get pulled over in the carpool lane. This was a little different, however, because we brought the dogs with us. Even so, Kate had to stay to feed the horses since we weren't sure when we would be back.

Georgia was there waiting for us when we arrived, and learned with us that this surgery involved contouring the new breast and making a new nipple from the skin that had replaced the original nipple. Dr. Da Lio was very pleased with the results from the first surgery and, I must say, I agreed. The new breast was nothing short of amazing and, except for the flat patch of skin where the nipple should have been, it looked perfect. He felt that it needed virtually no contouring and only the nipple formation. This surgery would take about an hour, Chris would be fine the very next day, and he wanted to do it the week before Thanksgiving. That worked fine with the schedule; it would be finished before I left for Africa, and also in time for her radiation treatments to begin on schedule for December 3rd.

After the appointment we walked, with the dogs, to the UCLA campus. UCLA was Georgia's alma mater and she knew of a place in the Student Union where we could get lunch and eat outside. The campus was alive with Monday activity and the two black Standard Poodles created quite a stir as we walked along. I waited outside with the dogs as Chris and Georgia went in to get lunch. At least ten girls stopped to gurgle and giggle at the sight of the dogs, and wanted to pet them. (There's a trick I wish I had known about in college... hang around with dogs to meet lots of women! Maybe in my next life...)

One of the girls was walking by, talking out loud to herself, when she spotted the dogs. She stopped walking, waited a second, then said, "Okay. There are two beautiful poodles here that I have to say 'hello' to; I'll talk to you later!" She hadn't been talking to herself after all, but had been on a cell phone with an earpiece that I hadn't seen! I laughed out loud.

Chris, Georgia, and I had a nice "picnic" lunch on the lawn, and the dogs were very well behaved and minded us, never running away or bothering anyone. It was great fun.

October 24:
6th (and Final) Chemo Treatment

The day of the final chemotherapy treatment had finally come. It was amazing that it had all gone so quickly, considering that it seemed like we were facing an eternity when we started in July.

Once again, Kate worked so she could take care of the animals and we did the usual driving routine.

And, happily, once again Georgia met us there.

This time, though, Chris felt a little apprehensive ("freaked out" was the term that she used) and she selected a treatment area that was about as far away from the previous areas as possible. Frankly, I was surprised that she hadn't felt that way any of the other five times she had been there. She likened this last treatment to a "black-diamond run," referring to the most difficult of the trails at a ski resort.

I was getting ready to get Thai food, but Chris told me she wasn't very interested in having any. She had suddenly developed an aversion to it due to its new association with chemo treatments; an aversion she still has to this day. It's a shame because she used to really like Thai food. In retrospect, we should have varied the food so she would not have developed any specific associations with the treatments.

I walked across the street and ordered food for Georgia and myself, then went to find a one-time use camera because I hadn't been able to find our own camera and we needed to have photos of this momentous last chemo-event. I ended up at St. Johns hospital, which was about two blocks away and, much to my delight, they did have a camera… and flowers, too. Duh… I hadn't even thought of that, this being Chris's last chemo and all.

With flowers and camera in hand, I went back to the Thai restaurant. When I walked up to pick up my food from the young Thai girl behind the counter, she saw the flowers and got all flustered, turning very red. As it turned out, she thought for some reason that they were for her and she didn't know what to do or what to say in her limited English. The young man that was working the counter with her explained it all and we had a good laugh. I picked up the food and then managed to carry everything back to the treatment room without dropping anything.

Chris definitely appreciated the flowers, although she was having a difficult time coping with this last chemo. The smell of the Thai food was making her sick, so Georgia and I ate quickly and disposed of the containers.

We were celebrating my upcoming birthday and Georgia gave me a CD that I had wanted. I realized I could play it on my laptop computer, so we listened to the CD while we were sitting there during the chemo. Then, in celebration of the last chemo and the new year to come, she also gave Chris a calendar with pictures of frogs in honor of "Marilyn," a toad that was living in our garden.

When that last drop of chemo poison went into Chris, Georgia, Iris, and I gave her a round of applause. It was finally over and we could leave this place for the last time.

As we began to leave, we overheard a conversation between a nurse and patient that clearly indicated that the patient was having her first treatment. Chris stopped to talk to her on the way out and told her that she was in really good hands and that she would love having no hair. "It's not so bad," Chris told her. "These treatments will be over before you know it."

When we walked out of the office, Iris told me, "Dave, you and your family have been an inspiration to all of us."

I was surprised to hear this. "Thank you for saying that, but why?" I asked her.

"Because of the love and support you have shown by being at all of Chris's treatments and always being in an 'up' mood. You wouldn't believe some of the things we see and hear around here."

In retrospect, the woman that Chris had just spoken to was alone and did look pretty dejected. Who could blame her? Chris probably would have been as well, except that Georgia and I kept her mind off of the treatments and kept her laughing. It is so important to be there. ALWAYS!

The previous treatment had been a few days after Georgia's birthday, and this treatment was a few days before mine, so Georgia treated us to a Japanese birthday dinner. We went to the same place we had gone for Georgia's birthday dinner, and had another exceptional meal. A plus was that the food was not the least bit spicy so Chris was able to eat it comfortably, even with her mucositis. We were all relieved that this phase of Chris's treatment was over, but that was easy for Georgia and me to say; Chris still had a week of feeling miserable ahead of her.

All of the prior treatments had been about the same (let's use "day 1" for the day of the treatment): day 2 Chris felt fairly normal, the evening of day 3 she would come crashing down and stay pretty much immobilized for days 4 and 5. On day 6 she would begin to come out of it and slowly start regaining her energy.

This treatment was different.

She never really did crash. Although she was weak, it was nothing like before when it was all she could do to get out of bed, go to the bathroom, and get back into bed. I'm happy to report that the last chemo left her with the easiest recovery.

Sunday (day 4) we cuddled on the couch and watched the 7th game of the World Series, which was very unusual for us because we never watch sports. It was the first time Chris had watched an entire baseball game EVER. There had been a lot of hype about it because it was between the California Angels (based in Anaheim, the closest major league team to us) and the San Francisco Giants and it had been a very exciting series. Since it was the last game, we started watching and got hooked. It was a nice moment, a first for us.

On the morning of my birthday (day 6) I didn't even realize what day it was until I heard Katie Couric mention the date on the Today show. I crawled into bed with Chris, who was just waking up. We talked for a while and she didn't mention what day it was. Then she decided that she was going to make pancakes from scratch; she just felt like it. We were in the kitchen and she was putting the ingredients into the mixer when she suddenly shook violently and yelled out, "It's your birthday! I'm sooooooo sorry that I forgot; I didn't even realize it! You don't deserve that..." and then she gave me a big hug. She ran out of the room and returned with a wonderful birthday card that she had purchased and prepared in spite of everything she had been dealing with.

A couple of months earlier she had asked me what I wanted for my birthday and I didn't really have any ideas. I am very hard to buy for because I really have just about everything I need, but I did come up with something, although it was relatively expensive. I told her that I wanted a new flat-screen monitor for my computer, which would enable me to sit at the return on my desk and drastically improve the comfort of my work environment. We discussed it and we agreed that she would get it for me and that it would count toward my birthday and Christmas, plus Valentine's Day and Father's Day of the following year. I actually purchased the monitor at that time and had had it several months by now, so I thanked her again for my birthday gift.

Usually for my birthday, Chris takes me to a movie, dinner, and then another movie, which is just about my favorite thing to do. She wasn't feeling all that well and felt badly that we wouldn't be able to do that. It was a little disappointing, although I certainly understood. That's okay, though; she would owe me!

The next Saturday night Chris decided she wanted to take me to dinner because I had been such a good caregiver. We went to a nearby restaurant and were having a nice meal and enjoying each other when I crunched down on something while chewing. A temporary crown, which I had gotten the day before Chris's last chemo treatment, decided to come loose. Fortunately it did not break and I went into the bathroom and put it back in using some Vaseline that Chris had had in her purse. (What's going to be next on this ride??) I ate the rest of my dinner carefully, to say the least. I was glad that I hadn't swallowed it!

The following day I had to deal with a sick horse. Keno wasn't feeling well; I could tell by the way he was acting and the fact that he wasn't eating, which is always a sure sign (especially with him!). I called the vet and she told me to give him some pain medication mixed in with some bran, and that seemed to do the trick. Right then and there I decided that I needed a night out, so Sonia and I went to dinner and then to a movie. Guess what came out during dinner? ...and broke when I accidentally bit down on it? I called the dentist from the movies but couldn't get hold of him, so I just had to wait until the next day.

Monday morning arrived and now I had a sick dog to deal with. When we went on our morning walk in the forest, Emma had diarrhea so I had to come back home, get a plastic bag, and "collect" a specimen. I took it to the vet and they found nothing wrong, but gave me antibiotics for her anyway. I got back just in time to take Chris over to Dr. Win so she could get her surgical clearance for the reconstruction surgery. I had learned my lesson from the mistake I had made before the big surgery in June, and this time I was doing it right by getting Dr. Win to fill out the form beforehand. As always during her chemo treatments, we were concerned about Chris being around others because of the germ factor, especially in a doctor's office where it isn't unusual to find lots of sick people. They let us in through a back door and right into an exam room so we could avoid all of that.

I grabbed some lunch and then went to the dentist, where they installed the permanent crown that, fortunately for me, had come in a day earlier than originally scheduled.

It was about this time that we received a renewal notice in the mail for a nutrition newsletter that we have received for years. I asked Chris if she wanted to renew and she told me to give her the renewal notice. She brought it back to me a few minutes later with a note she had written on it:

"I've always loved your newsletter and followed what it said. I got breast cancer anyway. So, now I don't read any health material and I eat pie. Thanks anyway, Chris Balch"

I laughed out loud. "You want me to send this??"
She said, "Yes, send it just like that!"
I did, and we haven't heard from them since.

November 12: 2nd Stage Reconstruction

Originally, Dr. Da Lio had told us that he would do the 2nd stage reconstruction surgery the week before Thanksgiving, but scheduling complications caused it to be moved a week earlier to a Tuesday. Chris has a standing appointment with Kim, her extremely busy and popular manicurist, every other Tuesday, so when I told Chris of the rescheduling, her first reaction was, "That's not a day I get my nails done, is it?" Geez! I guess we all have our priorities!

The new date was fine with us because it left more breathing room for scheduling the radiation appointments. This day's festivities were scheduled for noon (we had to be there an hour earlier), but they also wanted a cardiologist to do some tests on her heart because she was given Adriamycin as part of her course of chemotherapy. It seems that it has the potential, although quite unlikely, to cause a heart problem and they wanted to double check before administering the anesthetic. The cardiology appointment was at 9:15, so we had to leave pretty early.

Once again, Chris couldn't eat or drink anything for eight hours prior to surgery, so I got up about 3:30 to make sure that Chris ate something before the 4:00 a.m. deadline. I went back to bed for about 45 minutes, then got up to prepare for a 6:00 a.m. departure. By the time I fixed and ate my own breakfast, showered, walked the dogs, fed the dogs, and fed the horses, we just barely got out on time.

I would have preferred that we spend the night in the city so we wouldn't have to get up so early, but Chris really wanted to be home, so we toughed it out and drove in through the heart of Los Angeles during the worst part of rush hour on a Tuesday morning. I was expecting the worst, but it actually wasn't all that bad since we were able to use the carpool lane. It wasn't until we were within 4 miles of the hospital that the traffic became unbearable, especially considering that we were close to our time deadline. There was a considerable amount of stress during that last few miles.

Then, wouldn't you know it, we got behind a lazy driver. He changed lanes unexpectedly without signaling, didn't respond promptly when the light changed from red to green, and was driving much too slowly. To make matters worse, he ended up going into the same parking lot that we were, so the aggravation continued. Then, he was in the wrong lane, so he blocked our lane while waiting for an opening in the lane he wanted! Normally these things are merely annoying, but we were extremely tight on time and I was having a fit.

When I finally got around him, someone suddenly backed out of a space and almost hit us... was it just me or was everything working against us that morning??

We checked in at the cardiologist about 5 minutes late, which is remarkable considering the distance and the fact that it was us! The test turned out just fine, although it was pretty strange to see my wife's heart beating in three dimensions on a computer monitor.

We emerged from the office and Georgia was waiting for us. It was only about 9:45 so we had about 90 minutes to kill before reporting upstairs for the surgery. I wanted to stop at another office in the building because a few days earlier a friend of mine at the Los Angeles Chapter of the National Speakers Association told me she thought she had left a book there. I told her of our appointment and that I would stop by to see if they could find it. They looked and looked but never found the book, so we went to the lost and found for the building; it wasn't there either, but it served to pass some of the time. It was 10:15 and Chris suggested that we go to the surgery suite anyway; perhaps they could take her early.

We did and they did! Dr. Da Lio was running ahead of schedule and they were glad we were early. The only prob-

"... there is still life after chemotherapy and reconstructive surgery."

lem I could see was that, if they took her early it would be less than 8 hours since she last ate. When the anesthesiologist arrived at her bedside, I asked him about it and he said it wouldn't be a problem. (Actually, when he first arrived he asked what she had for breakfast. I told him, "A couple of eggs, hash browns, and two sausage links"... and then laughed. He said, "You know how bad it is to joke about taking a bomb on an airplane? I'll send you guys packin' in about two seconds!" and we all had a good laugh.)

They started the anesthetic and I got a little teary-eyed, but nothing like the two previous surgeries. I guess I was getting used to it. When they wheeled her off, Georgia and I walked to the same deli where we had had breakfast with Sonia the morning of the big surgery in June. After lunch we walked to a nearby grocery store to get some provisions for the drive home. By the time we returned to the surgical suite Chris was awake and just about ready to go; the procedure had gone better than they expected and was finished early.

We left and were on the road by 1:50, home by 4:00, and one more surgery (hopefully the last) was behind us.

The next day Chris was up early, made her own breakfast, did the laundry... she was amazing. She was able to do all of her normal activities (except anything strenuous), so all I really had to do was walk the dogs, feed the horses, and go on manure patrol. That gave me lots of time in the office.

The following Saturday we decided to go off-roading in the 4Runner on some of the nearby forest roads. We found a spot far away from everything and had a fun picnic with the dogs. Some of the roads are incredibly rutted and difficult to navigate but we managed, roaring along at 5 miles an hour.

As you can see, there is still life after chemotherapy and reconstructive surgery.

November 18: Dr. Da Lio Post Operative Appointment

Kate worked so she could take care of the animals, and we left early. The appointment was at 2:00 but we were going to meet Georgia for lunch at noon and had to drop off the 4Runner to be repaired, so we headed down to the city in two cars; I was in the 4Runner, Chris was driving the two-seater sports car (the "Z"). When the 4Runner was all tucked away in the repair shop and the service order was in place, we left for UCLA in the Z.

The Z is a much more powerful car than the 4Runner (lots of fun to drive, I might add), but it isn't nearly as comfortable. There is no place for Chris to lie down to sleep, so she had to make do with a reclining bucket seat and, needless to say, there wasn't any room for dogs.

We arrived only a few minutes late to lunch, and afterwards we rode over to UCLA in separate cars. We wanted to give Dr. Da Lio a thrill, so Chris brought along her fruit-hat. They showed us to the examination room and Chris undressed, put on her little hospital gown... and then the hat. And we waited.

The door opened and in came Dr. Da Lio, looking down at Chris's chart in his hands. When he looked up and saw the hat, the look on his face was priceless. He actually burst out laughing and looked at the hat in amazement, reaching out to touch it.

"You don't really wear that thing out in pubic, do you?" He was incredulous.

"Absolutely," Chris told him.

"She wore it to Costco," I said proudly. "She has had a lot of fun with that hat!"

He was in shock; I know he really liked the hat, and that he was impressed that Chris had the courage to wear it. At the mention of Costco he just looked at the floor and shook his head in disbelief.

Chris told him, "You've got to have as much fun with this as possible; the alternative is unthinkable."

It was great fun. Then she removed the hat so we could get down to some more serious business.

Dr. Da Lio removed the surgical dressings and we all admired Chris's new nipple. It looked just like the original, except for the color; it was simply amazing. The coloring for the nipple and areola was to be applied by way of a tattoo, the application of which is apparently a specialty. He told us that the woman in his office who did that sort of thing was no longer working there, and they had no one else in the office that could do it for her.

"We do have a woman we can refer you to, but she is very expensive and doesn't accept insurance," he told us as he was removing a few stitches. "I think you would be better off to go to the 'Black Wave,' a regular tattoo parlor on Santa Monica Boulevard. They do a good job and aren't very expensive as long as you don't get too fancy."

An unpleasant but amusing image leapt into my mind of a bunch of bearded, burly biker-types wearing leather vests standing around watching one of their own tattooing color onto my wife's nipple. I suppressed a laugh.

"How are they going to get 'Momma Never Loved Me' into such a small area?" I asked, trying to make it sound like an

---

"I doubt that he saw very many patients that laughed about the things they were going through as much as we did, but what else can you do?"

---

innocent question. "I guess they could make it a one-eyed eagle, couldn't they?"

We all started laughing and the jokes started flying. Chris thought the idea of going to a tattoo parlor was hilarious, and the three of us (Chris, Georgia, and I) were immediately looking forward to this event, which would be about six months after the radiation treatments were over; that would make it about the middle of July according to my rough calculation.

I honestly think that Dr. Da Lio didn't quite know what to make of us. I doubt that he saw very many patients who laughed about the things they were going through as much as we did, but what else could we do? The alternatives to laughing aren't very pleasant and there's nothing you can do about it anyway, so you might as well have as much fun with it as possible.

Dr. Da Lio left and I told Chris, "C'mon: get dressed, grab your hat and your new nipple, and let's get out of here."

Except for the follow-up Oncology appointments for the next 9 years, this ended Chris's treatment at UCLA. Since we knew we wouldn't be back anytime soon, we thought we would see if wonderful Dr. Brooks was in her office so we could stop by and say 'Hello'; besides, Chris wanted to show off her new breast and nipple. As we walked across the street to the hospital, Chris decided to wear her hat and we got lots of amused looks from passers-by, and some photos as well. Dr. Brooks was happy to see us and we were pleased to see that the photo we sent her, taken in pre-op just before the mastectomy/reconstruction, was displayed on a ledge in her office.

Georgia had parked in a lot nearby so we drove her to her car. This sounds much more normal that it actually was because we were in our 2-seater! Fortunately, Georgia is a small lady and she basically crouched in the footwell between Chris's legs for the four-block ride. She had to keep her head in Chris's lap so she couldn't be seen by any passing police, or I would have gotten a whopper of a ticket, I'm sure. One more little adventure in the context of the big adventure.

Chris and I hit the freeways at 4:00, the worst possible time of day on the most congested part of the most congested freeway in the world. Three hours later we were about half-way home so we stopped at one of our favorite restaurants and had a great meal. The rest of the ride home was an hour, just about what it was supposed to be, and we got home around 9:00.

...but the day wasn't over yet...

As Chris was getting ready for bed, she noticed something sharp sticking through her gown under her right arm. I looked and discovered, much to my dismay, that it was a stitch. IT WAS A STITCH! A stitch that Dr. Da Lio apparently missed because of all of the talking and carrying on about the tattoo parlor. Oh, great... another medical procedure for Nurse Dave.

I found a pair of small scissors that had a fairly sharp point, which I would need in order to get the scissors between her skin and the stitch itself. I thought I had snipped it, but when I pulled on it it wouldn't come out. The scissors weren't "pointy" enough. I couldn't get it. I considered just yanking it out, but decided that was a bad idea. (It was, in fact, a VERY bad idea!)

Messing around with the stitch was starting to get painful for Chris, so we decided to wait until morning and call our neighbor Kathy. Being an ER nurse she HAD to know about these things and have the right tools, too.

The next morning we completely forgot about the stitch and went about our business. Chris was very busy vacuuming and working around the house, and I had a conference call with my Internet marketing mentor and several of his other clients. They pretty much told me what I already knew, which was that the book I had been trying to market on the Internet wasn't going to sell and I should focus my efforts elsewhere.

I was devastated, but I knew they were right. I shed more than a few tears of disappointment, fear, and frustration over that one, but then I decided I would regroup and do something else; I just didn't know what.

The next day was also fairly normal, with Chris doing as much as she could and me doing my usual animal chores. It was about 8:30 that night that I suddenly remembered the stitch, and I had a physical reaction. When I took a look, I was horrified to see that the skin around the stitch had almost completely grown over it, and I was concerned that it was too late to remove it properly and that someone (not me!) was going to have to do something unpleasant to Chris in order to get it out. I couldn't bear it; she's been through enough, dammit.

We immediately called Kathy who, thankfully, was home. She came right over with her surgical scissors, climbing the fence between our homes and walking down a steep hill in the dark before I had a chance to go out there with a flashlight and meet her.

She came in the house, took a look at the stitch, snipped, pulled, and it was done. No pain, no fuss, no muss. I was so relieved!

November 21:
Radiation Consult/Simulation

Now that Chris's treatment at UCLA was complete, it was time to begin the "Loma Linda Adventure" for radiation therapy. It's kind of funny, really, when I look back at how scary it was starting up at the first hospital; so many new faces, buildings, procedures, etc. It wasn't long, though, until we knew our way around the facility and felt right at home. Then, when we switched to UCLA, we went through that whole process again, until we got familiar with new facilities and people there. Now it felt like we were being yanked out of that now-comfortable environment and were starting all over again with yet another new institution. Chris and I discussed this phenomenon, and the fact that we would soon know our way around Loma Linda and would no doubt feel right at home there as well.

When we started talking about it we realized that there was even another level to that cycle and that was the treatment regimens. The big surgery was scary, naturally, and dealing with the aftermath was too. But we fell into the rhythm of emptying drains, taking pain pills, my bathing of Chris, and all of the other new and strange activities, and when it was over we sort of missed it. Then came the chemotherapy lifestyle, including the regular appointments and their aftermath; once we settled into that routine, it wasn't so bad.

Now chemotherapy was over and a new chapter was beginning: radiation, and a whole new slew of people, places, medical terms, and questions. We knew that we would get used to this lifestyle as well, and that we would also love everybody involved.

> "It goes to show how adaptable we all are, and how unnecessary it is to fear the changes. It's hard *not* to fear them, but it is unnecessary nonetheless."

It goes to show how adaptable we all are, and how unnecessary it is to fear the changes. It's hard *not* to fear them, but it is unnecessary nonetheless.

Dr. Chap had wanted Chris to get a bone density test, which we were lucky enough to schedule just before the radiation consult which, in turn, had been combined into a single appointment with the simulation, which would be followed by a CT-scan. So today was a quadruple-whammy: four appointments combined into a single trip down the mountain.

Just before we left for the day's appointments, I got some very bad news from the Toyota dealer. It was going to cost another $1,900 to fix the 4Runner. I could feel my body deflate with despair; how the heck can I afford that? I realized that even if we sold that car and bought another one, I was going to end up paying for it anyway, so there was no easy solution. I told them to go ahead; it would be ready in about two weeks, which was getting dangerously close to my departure for Africa. It was critical that Chris have the 4Runner while I was gone because it was our only 4-wheel drive vehicle and she would need it if it snowed. They assured me that it would be ready by then.

The bone density test was easy compared to a lot of other things that Chris had been through. She changed into a gown, disappeared for about 10 minutes, and it was over. We waited another 10 minutes while the radiologist read the films and gave us the report, and we were on our way.

To be technically correct, Chris was being treated in the Radiology Department of the Loma Linda University Medical Center, in Loma Linda, California. It is 27 miles from our home, which translates into a 45-minute drive. Again, the reason we did not get radiation therapy at UCLA was the distance involved, coupled with the fact that we knew that radiation treatments were given every day, Monday through Friday, for six weeks. At two hours each way in good traffic, that would have been way too much driving, so the search was on for a closer treatment facility. We selected Loma Linda University Medical Center because of its world-class reputation; we are just lucky that it also happens to be just about the closest such facility to us anyway.

We arrived at the Radiation Department on time, and were greeted by Dr. Grover who looked very young. He was a resident and spent some time with us asking questions about the history of her cancer and treatments. Then Dr. Hocko, the radiologist, arrived and we explained everything again.

The two doctors examined Chris and, all told, spent about an hour with us. Then it was time for the simulation, so we went down the hall to a small room that contained a large machine. Chris had to get up on a table and they proceeded to calculate exactly what the machine settings would be and exactly what position she had to be in. It took about 45 minutes, and Chris had to lie there with her arm raised over her head, which became pretty darned uncomfortable after a while. I only know this because she told me; I was invited to leave the room before they began.

I was pretty hungry because we hadn't had time to get any lunch, so I went to the hospital cafeteria. It was there that I discovered that Loma Linda University Medical Center was a Seventh Day Adventist institution and, as such, was strictly vegetarian. Not even fish. And no caffeine, either, which meant no coffee and no tea except herbal tea. Also on the list of prohibited foods: pepper. I got a bowl of lentil bean soup for myself and vegetable soup for Chris. I was worried that she might have a sugar problem during the simulation, so I had told the doctors and technicians about it and that her honey was available, just in case.

When they let me back in the room, there she was with her arms in restraints at a weird angle above her head. She looked so helpless my eyes teared-up and I went over to her and stroked her head. She was almost in a trance... it was scary.

They had used a felt-tip pen to draw various marks on her skin to be used when positioning the machine for her treatments. Clear adhesive strips covered the marks so they would not be washed away when Chris showered, and they showed me how to re-draw and re-cover the marks in the event that any of the strips came loose and the marks began to fade. The technicians would make sure that the marks were legible during the treatments; it was more likely I would need to do this on the weekends when Chris wouldn't be seeing them.

When we finished, Chris ate her soup and we went down the hall and around the corner for the CT-scan, but the machine wasn't working so they asked if we could come back the next day. Since we were already in the city, we ran some errands and Chris took me out to dinner because I spent my entire day with her. We talked a lot about the bad news I had received that morning about the car repair, and decided that we simply could not afford to get a new car. Toyotas are incredibly reliable and we shouldn't have too much more trouble after this big repair, for a while at least. We know someone that has over 250,000 miles on their 4Runner and never even had this particular problem.

The next day we came back to Loma Linda for the CT-scan. They let me in the room while they were setting everything up, so I was able to hold Chris's hand and stroke her cute little bald head. As I left, I looked over my shoulder and saw her lying there, looking so helpless and at the mercy of yet another large machine, and it just broke my heart.

November 25:
Dr. Chap Follow-up

It's a good thing that I like to drive. We were going once again to UCLA for what we hoped would be our last visit for a while.

It was the usual scenario: Kate came in late and worked so she could take care of the animals. Chris and I took the Z because the 4Runner was still being repaired, although on this trip I didn't have to worry about being pulled over in the carpool lane because there was no place for Chris to hide in the 2-seater while she was sleeping.

We met Georgia for lunch at the deli and then took two cars over to the oncology offices, where we saw Dr. Chap for Chris's first post-chemo follow-up appointment. This was merely a check-up to make sure that there were no issues or questions about Chris's condition.

We found out that we would be seeing Dr. Chap every three months for three years, then every six months for two years, and then once a year after that.

We asked when Chris's hair would begin growing back in, and she told us that six to eight weeks after the last chemo treatment we should start seeing some "fuzzies." Seeing as how it had already been four weeks since the last treatment, she only had a couple of weeks to go!

Dr. Chap was such a delight: about half of our time together was spent chit-chatting about our lives. She gave Chris a hug and we were on our way, feeling good all over again about UCLA in general and Dr. Chap in particular.

I had a meeting of my Mastermind group that night in Pasadena, which is about 45 minutes from UCLA. Due to the distances involved, it was impractical for me to take Chris home and then drive to the meeting, so she came with me.

Although I had been a member of this group for over two years, Chris had never been to one of the meetings or met most of the members. So I was proud to show her off to my friends and colleagues.

Chris seemed to be back to normal by now, except that she got tired fairly quickly and needed a nap in the afternoon. Other than that, she was up and around doing her normal activities including spending time with her beloved horses. She even went riding a few times with Kate.

She still could not do any of the heavier chores having to do with the horses, such as picking up the manure and filling their feeders, but she did as much as she could because she likes being independent.

In the meantime, I was rushing around getting ready for my trip to Africa. Seeing her as active and healthy as she was, I felt less guilty than I thought I would. I had a lot to do before I left, including writing three articles for my newspaper column and preparing a newsletter to go out while I was away.

I was scheduled to leave at 11:55 p.m. Thanksgiving night, so Chris, Gail, Sonia, and I found a restaurant that was open and we went there for a nice dinner. I left from there for the airport and Gail and Sonia took Chris home.

Two days later, Georgia came up to the house to stay with Chris for a few days, and they were joined by John who drove down from Northern California. The three of them had a great weekend together. John and Georgia stayed on so they could go with Chris to her first radiation treatment the following Tuesday.

December 3:
Radiation Begins

Georgia, John, and Chris arrived at Loma Linda University Medical Center on time for the first radiation treatment. Just as the chemotherapy was designed to kill any errant cancer cells that had escaped from the tumor and entered the body through the lymph system, the radiation was designed to kill any cancer cells that might still be in the area near the original tumor.

Each of the 30 treatments was quite simple and straightforward; she would come into the radiation waiting room and change into a gown. They would call her in and position her on the table and then position the machine, which then ran for about a minute and a half. Then they would reposition the machine and run it again for about 30 seconds. After that, she would get off the table, change out of the gown, and leave. The total elapsed time from putting the gown on to taking it off was about 15 minutes.

And so it went every day, Monday through Friday, for the next six weeks except for Christmas and New Year's Day.

I returned from my trip on December 10 and drove directly from the airport to Loma Linda. The timing was perfect, and I arrived just a few minutes before she did. We were very happy to see each other, and went out for an early dinner after her treatment.

We had a lot to talk about! She told me that she was absolutely fine the entire time I was gone, and that the timing had been perfect since she had felt the best she had felt in a long time. I told her about my trip in gory detail, including the fact that it had been cloudy at the critical moment and we didn't get to see any part of the eclipse. Bummer, to say the least. The rest of the trip, though, had been spectacular and was just the get-away that I needed.

The radiation treatments were the first appointments or procedures of any kind that I had missed since the diagnosis eight months earlier, but it hadn't really been necessary for me to be there; at least not as far as Chris was concerned. It simply became her "job" to go to these treatments, and she fell into a routine.

The first thing Chris had done was experiment with the routing to determine the most efficient way to get to the hospital. It was about 45 minutes each way no matter how she did it, but some routes had less traffic than others and were therefore more pleasant to drive. She finally came up with a very efficient and enjoyable route that even cut about five minutes off the time.

She also decided that, since the weather was cool, she would bring the dogs with her. They would stop at a park at the bottom of the mountain and then go on to Loma Linda for the treatment. The dogs waited patiently in the car for the 15 minutes or so that Chris was gone, and then they went to a new dog park on the way home, where Emma and Simone could run around and play with other dogs, and Chris could just sit there and watch, throwing a tennis ball occasionally for their (and her) amusement.

This was Chris's routine for the first 4 weeks or so. Her energy was good and the radiation treatments didn't hurt or seem to affect her except that the area being treated was getting red, similar to sunburn.

Every few days the pen marks on Chris's skin would begin to fade and I had to draw them back on using the felt-tipped pen they had given me at the hospital. I would then cover the marks with the special tape that they had given us for that very purpose.

December 17:
The Occupational Therapist

Today we would be presented with Chris's next health-related surprise.

In conjunction with the radiation therapy, Dr. Hocko had referred us to Occupational Therapy where we would be introduced to lymphedema, a condition potentially caused by the removal of the lymph nodes during the lumpectomy back in May. We had heard about this condition but didn't really understand it or its ramifications and we were here to find out. I had scheduled the appointment so we could go directly to Chris's radiation treatment when we were finished.

When we arrived, the first thing we had to do was register. A woman called us in and Chris sat next to her desk as the woman asked a lot of questions. She was busily typing Chris's answers into a computer when she asked Chris, "What's your religion?" Chris answered, "Any religion that likes pepper!" (She was referring to the fact that Loma Linda is a Seventh Day Adventist institution and they have a dietary restriction on pepper.) We all had a good laugh, then we went back to the waiting room.

Enter Kimberly Wood, Occupational Therapist. Slender, attractive, and bursting with positive energy, she collected us and took us to a treatment room where she proceeded to examine Chris and begin our education in lymphedema 101.

Lymphedema is a condition that results from poor circulation of the fluid in the lymph system and causes the arm to become swollen. Chris is susceptible to this condition because of the lymph nodes that were removed during the lumpectomy. The lymph nodes are responsible for pumping the fluid through the lymph system and, since some were removed, the fluid could possibly accumulate in Chris's arm causing the swelling.

One way to avoid this condition is regular massaging of the arm and chest, encouraging the lymph fluid to circulate in a slightly different manner thereby helping to reduce the swelling potential. She showed Chris some massage techniques and they practiced them together a few times. She also gave us some charts and instructions and told Chris that she would have to wear a special "compression sleeve" on her right arm whenever she was in an airplane. For the rest of her life.

Also, for the rest of her life, Chris has to be careful not to lift too much weight with her right arm: because of the lymph node removal, she can't lift more than 15 pounds with that arm.

Kim was a very strong and positive presence, bursting with life. As usual, we joked with her and the entire session was full of fun and laughter, despite the news that Chris would have to deal with this for the rest of her life.

We told Kim that, so far at least, Chris hadn't had any problems with swelling all through the big surgery in June, the chemotherapy, or the radiation. Kim said that that was a good sign for the future, but that Chris still had to be diligent and aware of her potential for this condition.

She gave Chris some "homework" and we made a follow-up appointment for several weeks later.

Radiation Continues

It was New Year's Eve when Chris told me that she was getting too tired to make the daily drive to radiation, so I drove her down there for the each of the final two weeks' treatments. In the process of being at the hospital every day, Chris had met John and Linda, a couple who had a daily appointment at a time very close to hers, but in an adjoining radiation room. John was being treated for prostate cancer and Linda was a very supportive wife, coming with him to every treatment.

They were a charming couple with a wonderful sense of humor, and we would laugh and carry on whenever we saw them, which, with few exceptions, was every day of treatment. We tried to find fun everywhere we went, and we certainly found it with them.

Chris had also become very attached to the technicians, all of whom were really sweet and kind people. In fact, one day in mid-December, we had had a snowfall and Chris filled a cooler with snow and brought it in with her as a surprise. (Loma Linda is in the valley below the mountain and I doubt that they have ever gotten snow there.) A snowball fight immediately broke out in the hallway and they had a grand time. One of their supervisors wasn't too happy at this development, but *his* supervisor happened to come in and started throwing snowballs himself, so he lightened up a bit.

Everyone at Loma Linda was always nice and friendly to me, and allowed me to go with Chris into the radiation room as they positioned her on the table and adjusted the machine. I usually stood next to Chris, trying to comfort her by holding her hand or stroking her head, and when they were ready we all left the room, closing a six-inch thick door behind us. (What the heck were they doing to my wife that we had to go behind such an intimidating door??) In retrospect, perhaps I was comforting myself rather than Chris by touching her as they prepared the machine; she had been through this many times before and didn't seem to be bothered by it. I like to think, though, that she liked having me there.

As the treatments continued, Chris's skin began to blister, crack, and scab over. The fifth week it was extremely uncomfortable for her, and we were experimenting with various pain medications. We still had some of the Ela-max cream, which had been so effective in easing the pain of her shingles, so we tried that as well but it only helped a little bit. I felt so badly for Chris and, once again, was terribly frustrated that I couldn't do anything to help her.

Each treatment made her discomfort a little worse, and it finally got to the point where she had the equivalent of a third degree burn on her breast. It looked extremely painful and I put the cream on it a couple of times a day, but it just had to run its course and would heal in the same amount of time as other third degree burns would heal.

The doctor had prescribed a special cream that didn't do much for the pain but which was supposed to help the skin heal more quickly. There was no way to tell if it actually did any good, but it was comforting to use it under the theory that it was helping.

At the end of the fifth week, treatment number 25, we thought that Chris would have to endure five more treatments on this incredibly burned area. We got a nice surprise, however, when we were told that the treatment area was going to be changed slightly to concentrate on the scars from the surgery, and that the larger area, which was so sore, would no longer be treated. That was a huge relief, even though they said that the burned area would continue to get worse for a few more days. It did.

Every Wednesday was a "doctor" day and radiation patients were supposed to stop by the doctor's office after their treatments. Chris never really felt the need to do that, except for the fifth week when the burn was getting so bad. The doctor told her that this type of burn was not unusual, although hers was on the severe end of the scale because her skin was so fair. Chris would just have to tough it out.

January 15:
The Final Treatment

Chris decided that, in honor of her final radiation treatment, she would wear her Carmen Miranda hat. Everyone got a big kick out of it, causing lots of laughs and chuckles. John and Linda were particularly amused, and they had brought their digital camera for the occasion. I asked Chris to lie on the radiation table with the hat on and took a photo with my own camera.

We sat with John and Linda for a while before they called Chris in for her treatment. They said their goodbyes and, as Chris went into the treatment room, I had an idea and pulled them aside to ask them to wait in the hall for a few minutes. They said they'd be happy to wait. When Chris was all positioned and we went behind "the door" for the first time, I told all of the technicians (there were usually 4 of them) that I had some friends waiting outside and that I would like everyone to give Chris a round of applause when she got off the table for the last time. They thought it was a great idea.

After the last cycle they went in to get her off the table. As she sat up, John and Linda came in and the seven of us (4 techs, John, Linda, and I) burst into a vigorous round of applause, cheering, yelling, and hooting. It was a very small room and the noise was considerable. Chris was surprised and sat there beaming, enjoying the accolade. It was a nice ending to yet another phase of her treatment.

It was over. 268 days, 6300+ miles of driving, 81 appointments, procedures, and tests, three surgeries, six chemotherapy treatments, and 30 radiation treatments. Done. Finished.

I distinctly remember walking out of Loma Linda after the last treatment with an incredible sense of satisfaction and accomplishment. I felt like we had really accomplished something special together: Chris had fought the battle of her life and I had helped her do it. We had done all we could do; all that was left were the follow-up visits with Dr. Chap for the next 9 years, the waiting to see if the cancer would return, and trying to think positive thoughts.

Chris still had a few weeks of discomfort ahead of her as the burns healed and she regained her strength. Every day it was a little better, though, and now the discomfort is just a bad memory; a bad memory that fades with every passing day.

Yes, there were some bad moments. Yes, Chris had some very uncomfortable periods during her treatment. But what we remember most is the laughter that we shared with the doctors, nurses, and other patients, and the support that we got from our family and friends. And I remember Chris's extreme bravery and positive attitude during the entire ordeal.

I like to think (and Chris agrees) that I had something to do with her positive attitude. By removing all stress and worry about things that were important to her, she had no worries to weigh her down. She could focus on the illness and kick it in the butt.

You, too, will get through this. The most important thing to remember is that the situation is only temporary. There is another side to that cancer door, and you will slam that door closed with the satisfaction of a job well done.

And your life together will continue, and you will be all the better for your experience.

I can tell you this without any reservations whatsoever: taking care of my wife for these nine months was the most rewarding, uplifting, satisfying, and meaningful thing I've ever done. My business suffered. Our finances suffered. I endured a lot of stress and did lot of unpleasant things I never thought

I'd have to do. But I would do it again in a heartbeat, because this is what life is about. This is what it is to be human.

I feel that I have achieved something that few will have an opportunity to achieve. If you find yourself faced with a similar situation, and I hope that you do not, be brave. Take a deep breath and tackle it head on.

You'll be glad you did. There is no feeling quite like it.

Author's note: through it all, I never had to do a single load of laundry. I knew how and was certainly willing to, but Chris insisted that she was going to do it. And she did. Go figure.

Epilogue I

It seems appropriate to share some relevant things that have happened since the end of Chris's treatment. It is now July, 2004, 27 months since her original diagnosis. That makes her a 2+-year survivor (according to Dr. Chap, the measurement begins with the date of diagnosis). As far as I'm concerned, though, I, too, am a 2+-year survivor. *"She survived the cancer. I survived taking care of her!"*

Here are some items of interest, in no particular order, that pertain to our story and which will resolve some of the questions I've been asked.

We did, indeed, go to Tahiti for 7 days in order to celebrate the successful end of Chris's treatments as well as our 20th wedding anniversary. Kate and her husband, Alan, literally moved into our home and took care of the entire menagerie so that we could go. We left 15 weeks after the final radiation treatment.

Not only did we stay in an overwater bungalow, *we stayed in one of the very bungalows in the resort pictured on the post card* that we had put on the refrigerator during the darker days of chemo.

We could watch the fish through a portion of the floor.

Chris enjoyed snorkeling in the lagoon from our bungalow's private landing.

We swam with sharks and manta rays.

It was sweet.

We wanted to do something really special for Kate, since she did so much and asked for so little in return. Since money was an issue, we used frequent flyer miles to purchase two round-trip air tickets in her name to anywhere in the

United States. She and her husband used them to go to New York City for their 10th wedding anniversary.

We also gave her a week in a condo near Vail, Colorado, which was in exchange for a week we already had on deposit from a timeshare that we used to own. She is going to use it to go skiing with her family this winter.

After Chris's strong association between chemotherapy and Thai food, it was over a year before she could even think of Thai food again. We have, however, gone to a Thai restaurant since then, so that association has faded.

Chris's hair grew back nicely and she soon rediscovered how much work it was to have longer hair. About two months ago she had it cut and she wears it short now. It looks terrific but, more importantly, she is happy to have less work to do every time she shampoos.

Chris has been having regular follow-up appointments with Dr. Chap every three months, including an exam and a blood test. So far, everything looks perfect. Georgia hasn't missed any of these appointments and Dr. Chap braces herself when she sees the three of us waiting for her because she knows it's going to be pretty lively!

We did get a scare, though, after one of her blood tests came back with some abnormally high readings. Just to make sure, though, she had another CT-scan which would have shown us if new cancers were growing anywhere in her body.

The test results were fine, but going through it amplified the worry generated by the blood test.

As it turned out, this blood had been drawn a few days after Chris had returned from a short trip to visit some friends in Mexico, and she was a bit dehydrated. Dehydration makes the blood more concentrated and any given amount will contain more of everything than it normally would. When that was determined, everything was back to normal.

I am proud and humbled to report that a special panel of The Susan G. Komen Breast Cancer Foundation has reviewed and approved *Cancer for Two.* It is now listed at **www.komen.org** in two categories: "Breast Cancer Patient Support" and "Significant Other's Support."

As a result of this experience, I have a new career! In addition to writing this book I founded The Patient/Partner Project, which is focused on "helping the patients by helping the partners." We offer free resources and services for patients and partners, including free progress reporting for family and friends and free email mini-courses.

The Patient/Partner Project joined the National Quality Caregiving Coalition (NQCC) of the Rosalynn Carter Institute for Human Development. In the course of that journey, I had the privilege of meeting former first lady Rosalynn Carter and presenting The Patient/Partner Project to her and the NQCC – I invite you to visit **www.ThePatientPartnerProject.org** to see a photo of us together.

I also offer speaking programs about dealing with family crisis for all types of audiences, including patients and partners, medical professionals, employees, and business organizations. If you know of a group looking for such a program, visit **www.ThePatientPartnerProject.org** and click on "Speaking" for details and contact information.

If you are currently going through a struggle with any type of cancer or know someone who is, we want to help. Please visit or refer **www.ThePatientPartnerProject.org** to use our free services, and to tell us via "feedback" what else we can do that would be helpful.

Epilogue II – Cancer for Two Two

In August, 2004, Chris had a mishap while horseback riding when her horse was crowded and forced so close to a tree that Chris hit it. She didn't fall off, but her knee and leg were caught and bent back as they passed. Naturally her hip was stiff and sore, but it didn't seem to be getting any better so she went to physical therapy. It still wasn't getting better so Sandy, her physical therapist, suggested that Chris have an MRI of her hip to see what was going on.

Again, it was Dr. Win who gave us the results.

"Your hip is broken," she told us, as our jaws hit the floor. "... *and that's the good news.*"

Uh-oh.

"The MRI shows evidence of cancer in your pelvis."

My tears came instantly. Oh, no... we had heard about cancer "metastasizing," which is when it spreads from its original location to other places in the body. But, once again, that is something that happens to other people, not to us. Chris had been getting blood tests every three months to catch this sort of thing before it spread too far, but the tests aren't perfect (duh) and don't catch some situations.

We called Dr. Chap over the weekend and by 10:00am Monday morning we had 4 appointments for various consults and tests. Two weeks later we got the news: cancer had spread throughout her skeleton, and there were spots on her skull and liver as well. (They did an MRI on her brain but didn't find anything... I told Chris that they wouldn't't!)

The broken hip put her in a wheel chair for 3 months. Radiation on her pelvis began immediately, as well as weekly infusions and a new round of chemotherapy (described later). Lots more driving, this time through the winter, which, as it turned out, was one of the wettest in our mountain community in 30 years. I can't even begin to describe all of the ramifications of that, but here are some examples. In one particular storm we got 18 inches of snow followed by 24 inches of rain in 3 days! During another storm, the top 35 feet of a 100-foot cedar tree snapped off in slushy snow and heavy winds and landed on the driveway, blocking us in until I could remove it. ...and on and on. (Remember, this is Southern California...)

On one of our weekly trips to UCLA we discovered to our dismay that all roads off our mountain were closed by mud and rock slides; it was impossible to get down to the city.

Unless, that is, you are Chris Balch on a mission.

Much to my horror, she decided to try driving down anyway and drove around one of the roadblocks. (We later discovered that was an even crazier thing to do than we had thought at the time because, in some cases, the roads were *completely* washed out... in other words, GONE.)

We made it almost all the way to the freeway before we encountered a Highway Patrolman who wanted to know how we got to where he had stopped us. As he approached the car I told Chris, "Take off your hat!"

She took off her hat, exposing her once-again bald chemo-head and told him that she had driven around the roadblock because she had to get to her chemo treatment.

Maybe I imagined it, but he first looked at her head then sounded very exasperated when he told us to go ahead, "but be careful and don't ever do that again!" (That's when we learned that sometimes the roads are washed-out...)

Chris was very worried (we both were) that this was going to be "it", so she made lists of her things and to whom I should give them if the worst happened. I was crying a lot of the time for many different reasons; this go-round was much harder for me because, *besides the fact that I could lose her:*

1) the weather was MUCH worse resulting in incredibly hard physical work as well as frustrating road closures (one night we couldn't get back home due to a washed-out road),

2) her wheelchair confinement meant she couldn't do as much as she did during the initial round of treatments,

3) we had to drive to UCLA *every week* for five months for the infusions (Herceptin and Zometa every week, plus chemotherapy every 3 weeks) and coordinate that with daily radiation for the first six weeks and

4) the money situation wasn't any better and now we had full deductibles to meet for both 2004 and 2005.

Because of her new schedule of weekly infusions, Chris needed a "port-a-cath." This is a device into which they can directly inject the infusions rather than starting a new IV each time. (This is important because a new IV every week is not only painful and difficult to do, but could permanently damage Chris's veins.) It was implanted in her upper chest wall, between her shoulder and breast, in an outpatient surgery. That makes four surgical entries on Chris's cancer résumé.

Her last chemo was March 3, 2005. *As of March, 2006 all tests show that the cancer is as good as gone. Everywhere. And her hip fracture has healed, too.* She is one tough cookie!

At this writing Herceptin is a relatively new drug, which seems to have made the difference by suppressing the growth of new cancer cells while chemo killed the existing cells. Zometa will help repair damage to her bones caused by the tumors.

We still go to UCLA every three weeks for Herceptin and Zometa, which will continue "until further notice." Plus, now that we know that the blood tests don't work for her, Chris will have periodic CT-PET scans and bone scans to make sure that she remains cancer-free.

She feels terrific now and is living her dream. She rides her horse every other day (bareback, no less), picks up all the, uh, "used hay," rakes and maintains the riding trails in the forest, and tends to our little apple orchard. She even planted and cared for a beautiful flower garden this year.

Once again, life is sweet.

Appendix 1:
"Chris-isms"

1. "On the roller coaster of life, it's my turn to be in the front car. "

2. "If you're going to be in the front car, you might as well try to enjoy it 'cuz you ain't gettin' off in the middle of the ride!"

3. "Bring it on; I've always wondered what I'd look like with no hair."

4. "Stay in the moment. Why not make the best of things, no matter what? Some things are just going to happen no matter how much you worry about them."

5. "Having cancer is the best excuse I've ever had. If there's something I don't want to do I can just say, 'I can't; I have cancer.'"

6. "I *am* a Cancer, I'm not supposed to *get* Cancer."

7. "Hair is highly overrated."

8. "I look at people like the families of the victims of 9/11 and realize that I don't have it so bad after all."

9. "People think that I'm so brave and have such a good attitude, but I'm the same person I've always been; it's just that nobody ever noticed."

10. "It was nine months from diagnosis to my final treatment, and I gave birth to a new boob."

11. "I am *not* my hair."

Appendix 2:
"Dave-isms"

1. "It was her job to get better. It was my job to do everything else."

2. "Don't go there 'til you get there."

3. "If you aren't happy with the care you are getting, there probably *are* options."

4. "Your life is going to be turned upside-down for a while: you will be stressed, appointments and scheduling will be chaotic, treatments and decisions will be complicated. There's nothing you can do except deal with it."

5. "Don't be afraid to challenge some of the rules; they may not be what they seem."

6. "Everything seems worse when you're tired."

7. "With a little creativity, it is possible to turn an unpleasant situation into something fun."

8. "The more you learn about something scary, the less scary it becomes."

9. "Juggling my life became my way of life."

10. "There is great comfort in knowing that you're on the right path, even if that path is a scary one."

Appendix 3:
Fascinating (?) Facts

From discovery of the lump (April 10, 2002) through the final radiation treatment (January 15, 2003):

Dave: weight gain from comfort food	25 lb
Dave: weight loss from worry and stress	24.5 lb
Chris: net weight gain	
Number of get-well cards	85
Number of emails from newsletter subscribers	183
Total paid by us – drugs (prescription and over-the-counter)	$ 683
Number of traffic violations (estimated)	127
Number of *tickets* for traffic violations	0

TOP SECRET

More fascinating (?) facts...

	Round 1 4/10/02 thru 1/15/03	Round 2* 10/15/04 thru 6/21/05	Treatment Total 4/10/02 thru 12/31/05
Number of months	9	8	45
Total billed medical expenses	$ 188,175	$ 219,694	$ 551,148
Contractual adjustments**	$ 107,525	$ 117,603	$ 303,689
Total paid by insurance	$ 73,698	$ 90,722	$ 227,651
Number of medical appointments	81	82	183
Our portion of medical bills	$ 6,952	$ 11,369	$ 19,808
Cost of meals related to treatments	$ 1,229	$ 1,255	$ 3,012
Total miles driven	6,391	8,308	18,155
Auto costs (@ $.36/mile)	$ 2,340	$ 2,991	$ 6,536
Total out-of-pocket cost	$ 10,521	$ 15,615	$ 29,356

* See Epilogue II – Cancer for Two Two on page 244.
** Reduction in billed expenses based on agreements between Blue Cross and medical providers.

Appendix 4:
Reasons Why Cancer Was a "Gift"

1. Chris went through the dreaded "cancer door" and it wasn't so scary on the other side.

2. Chris found out who her true friends were.

3. Chris got to hear her own "eulogies". People always say nice things about you after you die, but the problem with that is that you never get to hear them. She got to hear them because people told her how strong and brave and inspiring she was, and that she was so wonderful she didn't deserve this, etc.

4. We are closer now than we ever were. (I think it was the washing, drying, and styling of her hair that did it!)

5. We met a lot of nice people; not only doctors and nurses, but other patients as well.

6. Before her cancer, people asked Chris how she could eat some of the healthy things she ate, and she would always say, "Because I don't like hospital food." (The implication was that she didn't want to be in the hospital for some illness caused by improper eating.) She found out that hospital food is actually pretty good! (At least it is at the UCLA Medical Center...)

7. Chris loved having no hair – no shaving her legs, underarms, etc., for four months.

8. Chris discovered a new look after her hair grew back in – short, naturally colored hair.

9. Chris has more patience after the cancer than she ever did because she now realizes how unimportant so many things are.

10. Chris has more appreciation for life in general and for nature, the people, and the animals in her life in particular.

11. Chris found out that she was stronger than she thought she could be.

12. Chris learned that it really doesn't matter what people think of you, and not to care when others are staring.

13. It forced Chris to slow down.

14. I had the opportunity to experience the incredible satisfaction and joy of taking care of the most important person in my life.

15. We have new respect for each other: me for her because of the way she handled it, her for me because of the way I dropped my life and took such good care of her.

16. She owes me, big-time! (This is my crass, trying-to-make-a-joke-out-of-everything way of saying that I know that if I am ever in a situation similar to Chris's, she will do the same for me as I did for her.)

Appendix 5:
Good Things About
Having No Hair

1. Save money on razors: no shaving anywhere.

2. An empty drawer where your curling iron, hair dryer, and several different brushes were located.

3. Save on shampoo, cream rinse, hairspray, gel, mousse.

4. No need for a brush means one less thing in your purse.

5. Don't care if the windows are down in the car.

6. Don't have to use deodorant (not that she had to anyway...)

7. Since it takes less time to get ready, she is rarely late any more.

8. Save money on haircuts, color, and perms.

9. No loose hair on your clothes.

10. No bikini-waxes (yes, when you lose your hair, you lose *ALL* of your hair...)

Appendix 6:
Tips for the Part-Time Caregiver

I was lucky in that, working at home, it was relatively easy for me to juggle my schedule in order to go to appointments and to do as much as I did. Many, if not most, caregivers will not have that flexibility due to job-related responsibilities. These caregivers may therefore not be able to be the full-time caregivers they would like to be.

There are still a number of things that you can do as a part-time caregiver that will be very helpful to the patient. I have culled a number of things from my experience that apply equally to full- and part-time caregivers.

1. Your number one priority should be to remove or reduce every shred of stress from the patient so that she can spend all of her energy fighting the disease. Everything you do should revolve around that basic principle, *but "removing as much stress as possible" does not mean "do everything for her."* It all depends on your patient and what is stressful to her; having someone else do certain things for her may actually *in*crease her stress instead of reduce it. In our case, I wanted to do all of the driving so she could sleep, but she wanted to do some of the driving so she could feel like she had control over *something*; my insistence on driving caused her more stress than it saved her, so she did enough of the driving to satisfy that need, then I took over.

2. Make use of the free services on the Internet at **www.ThePatientPartnerProject.org** to post progress reports, and then give the web address and your unique Member ID to all of your friends and relatives so they can

stay updated without having to call you and cause undue stress on your time. (The system is completely private and secure: no one can read your reports unless they know your unique Member ID.)

3. Allow the patient to express herself without comment, recrimination, or criticism – it's not your responsibility to "fix" everything.

4. Try to find humor wherever you can, especially self-deprecating humor.

5. Remember "Don't go there 'til you get there" – there are some things over which you will have no control, so try not to even think about how you will deal with these things until you have to. In many cases, the things you feared will never come to pass anyway. The perfect example was my fear of danger and difficulty getting to daily radiation appointments because of winter weather. The weather never materialized and had virtually no affect during the radiation treatment period. Had I worried and fretted about that when I first realized the potential, I would have been wasting energy: there was nothing I could do about it anyway, and there was the very real possibility that it wouldn't be a problem in the first place. Focus on the things that you can control, not on things you cannot control. It's easy to say, but hard to do.

6. Everything seems worse when you're tired. The same is true of the patient, who will be tired a lot of the time. Try to remember this so that when you are feeling overwhelmed and discouraged, you can chalk some of it up to being tired. And, by reminding yourself that everything is worse when you're tired, you are also giving yourself hope by realizing that you will feel better after you've gotten some rest.

7. Don't do anything that will generate additional stress unless it is absolutely necessary. For example, this is not the time to decide to sell your home and move, which is a very stressful undertaking.

8. Give yourself and your patient something to look forward to, such as a vacation when the treatments are over. Spend time planning and talking about it. The anticipation will give you energy when you need it the most.

9. When your patient asks for something, not only should you do it, but tell her "I would be happy to do that for you." *And mean it.*

10. Take time to take care of yourself, including exercise and time away from the situation. You need your physical and emotional strength, so if you need to get away and go to a movie, do it. You *need* it, and you *deserve* it. As they say during the airline safety speech, "Put on your own oxygen mask before helping others with theirs."

11. Be protective, but not overly protective. Part of the suffering for the patient is the loss of control over her life, so if she wants to do something and it won't be harmful to her medical condition, let her; it will help her feel better about herself.

12. Tell her often how great she looks, *and mean it.*

13. Tell her often how brave she is, *and mean it.*

14. Don't always trust how you feel; stress and anxiety can do strange things to your priorities and confidence, including feelings of overwhelm, hopelessness, and fear.

15. Don't take things personally. Her reactions and emotions are based on how she is feeling, which is pretty lousy a lot of the time. If she gets overly emotional or snaps at you about something, it is probably due more to the way she feels than to anything else.

16. Her desires may seem impractical, but you do them for *her* rather than for the reason she says. For example, Chris would ask me to change the dog's water even though it looked pretty clean to me. It didn't really need changing in my opinion and my first reaction was annoyance at having to do something (anything) that wasn't necessary in my view, but *it made her feel better* so that was the reason I did it.

17. She may feel ugly or unattractive, so do what you can to help her feel pretty, such as a manicures, pedicures, or special makeup.

18. You must be an advocate for your patient. If you don't like the care she's getting, *speak up*! If you don't understand something, *ask about it*! If you don't like the answers you're getting or the way you are being treated, *go somewhere else*!

19. Remember that you can handle more than you think you can. Things will come up that you don't think you can handle, but you will *because you have to*. Don't spend time thinking about how you can't handle something, just do whatever it is that you think you can't handle; you will surprise yourself.

20. Remember the pain of the current situation is only temporary. You're miserable for a while, and then it's over. Life WILL get back to some sort of normalcy. After all we

went through, what we remember most is all of the laughter we had.

21. You don't have to share *everything* with your patient. For example, my worry about the weather during radiation treatments that I mentioned earlier; why say anything about it? It could only upset her, nothing could be done about it at the time, and it may never happen.

22. People will offer to help in various ways, some of them will *insist*. Remember this about that:

- *It is not your responsibility to satisfy their need to help*. It is wonderful that they want to help and tell them that you appreciate it, but if what they are offering is not something you want or need, tell them "No, thank you." Well-meaning people can actually *increase* your stress rather than reduce it by insisting that you let them help: don't accept help you don't want or need. Be polite, but firm. I cannot overemphasize how important this is to your peace of mind and stress level. Don't be lulled into the trap of feeling guilty because you are not allowing them to do something they want ("need") to do. *Protect yourself from well-meaning but needy people*; you have your own needs to meet and they are far more important than theirs, especially now. It doesn't matter what your reasons are; if you don't want their help you don't have to accept it, and you don't have to explain why.

- Rather than simply saying "No," another way you can protect yourself is to thank them and say that you'll call when you need their help. For example, several people *insisted* on driving Chris to some of her daily radiation treatments and wouldn't take "No" for an answer. Chris wanted to drive herself to those treatments, and when she couldn't she wanted me to do it. So we simply told them we'd call them but never did. We truly appreciated their willingness to help and told them so. We simply chose not to take them up on it.

- The other side of this coin is that if people are offering help that you *do* need or want, *accept it.* We got many offers from friends who wanted to make food for us. My first inclination was to say "No," because I didn't want to be a burden to them and I didn't want to seem like I needed it. Guess what? I *did* need it. This was our time to accept the help that we needed, and providing meals was about the best thing that anyone could do for us in our particular situation. As far as being a burden, I took some of my own advice about that: "It's not my job to protect them from making an offer that they don't really mean, and it's not my responsibility if they end-up doing something they don't really want to do." We had several friends that went overboard in this particular area, but the food was great, they really wanted to do it, and they weren't pushy about it. Anne and Terry even went to one of our favorite restaurants on their way back home from the city and picked up some great meals, which lasted several days. God bless 'em!

23. Sometimes, due to lack of time or emotional energy you just won't feel like talking on the phone, even to caring and well-meaning people. If you don't feel like answering the phone, *don't.* This is your time to take care of yourself, not others; just because someone wants to talk to *you* does not obligate you to talk to *them,* so let them leave a voice message and return the call when you feel more like talking.

24. Take every opportunity to protect yourself from anything and everything that will cause you even the slightest additional stress or anxiety. If you are expecting an important call, screen your calls to save yourself from a conversation you don't feel like having. If you are unable to screen your calls and you answer a call for which you simply don't have time, tell them politely but firmly that you are expecting another call and you must leave the line open. Well-meaning people who truly care want to know what is going on, but your first responsibility is to your patient and to yourself and relieving yourself of any additional demands on your time.

Appendix 7:
Tips for Recording Doctor Visits

1. Use a small, portable recorder.

2. Always bring a fresh set of batteries, just in case. Even if the batteries are okay when you leave the house, it is possible that the recorder will be left on or start running accidentally while en route, which would drain the batteries before you arrive.

3. Record each appointment on a separate cassette... cassettes are inexpensive and it's worth the extra cost to be able to find something quickly.

4. Before you leave the house, load a fresh cassette into the recorder and make sure the batteries are okay so that you are ready to record without delay. If the doctor should come into the examination room earlier than expected, the last thing you want to do is unwrap a new tape and fumble around with the recorder. If you are talking to a nurse or someone that you didn't expect, mention their name so it is recorded on the tape as part of your record of the conversation.

5. When the doctor comes into the room, start the recorder first, then ask him/her out loud if it is all right that you record the visit. That way, on the tape, you will be able to hear them say it's okay. This will eliminate any potential controversy over whether you had their permission to record. If the doctor refuses, you must turn off the recorder and then, in my opinion, find another doctor. I would not trust a doctor who refuses to be recorded, and I certainly

don't trust my own memory to remember all of the details without error.

6. Remember the reason that you are recording: so that you can refer to the tape if you have any questions about what the doctor said about treatment, drug schedule, or instructions of any kind. You are NOT recording for potential legal action! Keep your eye on the ball here... remembering your intent will help keep you focused on ensuring that the important points are clearly recorded. If some important instructions are mumbled or you aren't sure if they recorded clearly, ASK THE DOCTOR TO REPEAT THEM 'FOR THE TAPE'.

7. Know where the microphone is and position the recorder as close to the doctor as possible in order to more clearly record his/her voice. Don't hold it in the doctor's face like a TV reporter – you don't want to be a distraction or an annoyance.

8. Label each cassette as soon as you get home with date, time, and doctor's name.

9. Remove the safety tabs from the cassettes so they cannot be re-used and erased by mistake.

10. Keep all of the cassettes together in a safe place so you can easily find them if you need them.

Appendix 8:
Tips for Reducing Stress

Both you and your patient will be experiencing new levels of stress and anxiety. Don't ignore them, but be proactive and do something about it. Here are some ways you can reduce your stress.

1. Drugs – no, I'm not talking about recreational drugs: there are many new anti-anxiety drugs available and I strongly suggest that you investigate your options. If you have a problem asking for this type of help, my advice is "get over it." Many people think that getting psychological help is shameful, but they are wrong. It is irresponsible, in my opinion, *not* to take advantage of the help that is out there, and these drugs can make the difference between night and day. There is no shame in getting the help you need, especially now when you need it more than ever. I personally know several people who suffered terrible anxiety, stress, and fear when they were diagnosed. They made appointments with a psychiatrist and were given "cocktails" of anti-anxiety medications that, literally, turned their worlds around.

2. Don't watch the news – the daily barrage of murders, fires, and traffic accidents is way too depressing and stressful when you're feeling well, let alone when the weight of the world is upon you.

3. Laugh – at anything and everything. If you are having trouble finding something in your situation to laugh at, read funny books and magazine, or rent movies that are comedies.

4. Go to movies – especially comedies.

5. Choose to avoid people that are negative or non-supportive. You need to spend your time with people who *reduce* your stress, not add to it.

6. Have something to look forward to – plan a vacation or a visit with family. The anticipation of the event will give you positive energy.

7. Try to remember that everything is worse when you're tired, so if you are feeling particularly down, remind yourself that you will feel better after you've gotten some rest.

8. Take time for yourself – whatever rejuvenates you. Take a walk, have dinner with friends, meditate, listen to music, etc.

9. Remember that the situation is only temporary.

10. Talk about how you feel with close friends/relatives.

11. Exercise.

Index

Adriamycin, 169, 170, 217
Amgen, 185
Ativan, 171, 172, 186
attitude, 21, 35, 121, 141,
    168, 187, 192, 239, 247

bears, 200
Big Bucks in a Bathrobe,
    ix, 51
biopsy, 17, 20, 24, 25, 26,
    32, 46, 61, 62, 64, 160
Blue Cross, 37, 38, 90
bone density test, 226
bone scan, 85, 89, 99, 100,
    104, 106, 107, 123, 164,
    166
Book Expo, 59, 60, 66
Brooks, Dr. Mai, xiii, 60,
    61, 62, 63, 64, 88, 89, 90,
    91, 93, 103, 106, 122, 123,
    127, 128, 144, 222

Carmen Miranda, 181, 194,
    238
Chap, Dr. Linnea, xiii, 122,
    123, 125, 163, 164, 165,
    166, 170, 171, 174, 176,
    183, 186, 194, 200, 226,
    229, 239, 241, 242, 244
chemo. *See* chemotherapy

chemotherapy, xiii, 54, 55,
    69, 83, 89, 92, 123, 124,
    146, 154, 164, 165, 166,
    167, 168, 170, 171, 173,
    174, 176, 177, 182, 183,
    185, 188, 189, 192, 193,
    194, 196, 198, 199, 200,
    202, 205, 206, 207, 208,
    209, 211, 212, 213, 215,
    217, 219, 225, 229, 231,
    234, 238
chicken pox, 181, 183
clean margins, 45, 73, 144
comfort food, 40, 109, 128,
    250
Compazine, 171, 172, 177,
    186
compression sleeve, 234
Costco, 153, 186, 193, 194,
    221
County Fair, 198
cranial prosthesis, 166, 174
CT-scan, 89, 106, 107, 108,
    123, 164, 166, 226, 228
cyst, 23, 160
Cytoxan, 169, 170

Da Lio, Dr. Andrew, xiii,
    91, 92, 93, 102, 103, 106,
    113, 121, 123, 125, 127,
    128, 129, 141, 153, 154,
    158, 159, 207, 208, 209,

217, 218, 220, 221, 222, 223. *See* Da Lio, Dr. Andrew

Dexamethasone, 176

diagnosis, x, 18, 32, 48, 49, 51, 54, 58, 63, 64, 164, 182, 232, 248

Dr. Janet Hocko. *See* Hocko, Dr. Janet

Dr. Kari Enge. *See* Enge, Dr. Kari

Dr. Kyi Kyi Win. *See* Win, Dr. Kyi Kyi

Dr. Linnea Chap. *See* Chap, Dr. Linnea

Dr. Mai Brooks. *See* Brooks, Dr. Mai

drain, 46, 75, 77, 78, 85, 100, 149, 150, 152, 153, 261

ductal carcinoma in situ, 26

eclipse
partial, 116
total, x, 116, 117, 136

Ela-Max, 183, 186, 187, 193, 194

Enge, Dr. Kari, xiv

family history, 64

Gel-Clair, 201

guided imagery, 97

hat party, 179, 180

Herceptin, 246

Hocko, Dr. Janet, xiv, 227, 233

hot flashes, 179

implants, 83, 84, 89, 92, 93

insurance, 20, 37, 38, 90, 101, 165, 166, 184, 186, 221

Loma Linda, xiv, 207, 225, 226, 227, 228, 231, 232, 233, 235, 239

lump, 17, 23, 24, 25, 27, 39, 45, 46, 64, 70, 73, 160, 250

lumpectomy, 45, 64, 88, 99, 105, 107, 144, 145, 146, 233

lymph nodes, 46, 73, 79, 83, 89, 123, 164, 167, 233

lymphedema, 233

mammogram, 32, 35, 39, 45, 64, 160, 161

margins, 73, 83, 166

mastectomy, 58, 83, 88, 90, 92, 100, 101, 103, 106, 119, 127, 128, 133, 222

metastasis, 244

Mohawk, 174, 175

mucositis, 200, 206, 213

multi-disciplinary conference, 106, 111, 112, 119, 120, 122, 125, 163 nausea, 165, 169, 171, 186, 195

Neulasta, 170, 172, 177, 185, 195

Oh, Canada, 79

Pac-Man, 97, 98
port-a-cath, 246

radiation, 20, 83, 84, 89, 92, 99, 123, 124, 154, 165, 189, 207, 208, 209, 217, 222, 225, 226, 227, 230, 231, 232, 233, 234, 235, 236, 238, 250, 255, 258
reconstruction, 83, 89, 92, 93, 101, 106, 119, 133, 134, 154, 158, 159, 206, 207, 209, 215, 217, 222
recording doctor visits, 29, 121, 166, 261
Revlon/UCLA Breast Center, xiii, 59, 63, 91, 102, 107, 120, 161, 163

second opinion, 58, 59, 61, 64, 88, 106, 123
sentinel node, 45, 46, 47, 64, 70, 73, 74
sentinel node biopsy, 45, 47, 64
September 11, 157, 191, 192

shingles, 181, 183, 184, 186, 188, 201, 236
simulation, 20, 97, 207, 208, 226, 227
Star Wars, 94, 96
Stay-at-Home CEO, ix, 28, 37, 51, 60, 66, 187
stress, 19, 20, 21, 40, 41, 42, 43, 49, 59, 60, 76, 81, 94, 95, 96, 119, 125, 137, 181, 183, 189, 199, 202, 208, 218, 239, 250, 254, 255, 256, 258, 260, 263, 264
survival rate, 84

Tahiti, 178, 180, 189, 241
Taxotere, 169
The Stay-at-Home CEO™, ix, 28, 51
therapy dog, 138
tissue expander, 84
total eclipses of the sun. *See* eclipse
TRAM-flap, 89, 90, 92, 102, 103, 106, 119, 158

UCLA, 59, 60, 61, 62, 88, 89, 90, 93, 101, 102, 103, 104, 105, 106, 107, 108, 111, 112, 120, 121, 124, 151, 163, 207, 208, 209, 220, 222, 225, 227, 229, 251

Valtrex, 188

wig, 166, 174
Win, Dr. Kyi Kyi, xiii, 17,
23, 24, 26, 27, 63, 112,
160, 161, 182, 188, 199,
215, 244

Zofran, 186, 195
Zometa, 246

CANCER *for* TWO

Quick Order Form

✂

INTERNET ORDERS: www.CancerForTwo.com

FREE E-BOOK for Internet orders: download the *Cancer for Two* eBook to begin reading right away, even while waiting for your printed book to arrive in the mail.

Fax orders: (909) 337-4945 (Fax this form)

Telephone orders: toll-free (800) 366-2347; use credit card

Postal orders: Cancer for Two
P.O. Box 824
Twin Peaks, CA 92391 USA

Please send _____ copies of *Cancer for Two* @ $18.95* each to (*please print clearly*):

Name:_____

Address:_____

City:_____State:_____Zip:_____

Telephone:_____

Email address:_____

Sales tax: We will add appropriate sales tax for books shipped to California addresses.

Shipping by air: We will add…
US: $5 for the first book + $2 for each additional book.
International: $10 for the first book + $5 for each add'l book.

Credit card type: [ ] Visa   [ ] MasterCard   [ ] AmEx

Card number:_____

Name on card:_____Exp. Date: ____/____

Signature:_____ ✂

* Quantity pricing available upon request

CANCER *for* TWO

Quick Order Form

INTERNET ORDERS: **www.CancerForTwo.com**
> *FREE E-BOOK for Internet orders:* download the *Cancer for Two*
> eBook to begin reading right away, even while waiting for your printed
> book to arrive in the mail.

Fax orders: (909) 337-4945 (Fax this form)
Telephone orders: toll-free (800) 366-2347; use credit card
Postal orders: Cancer for Two
P.O. Box 824
Twin Peaks, CA 92391 USA

Please send _____ copies of *Cancer for Two* @ $18.95*
each to (*please print clearly*):

Name:_____

Address:_____

City:_____State:_____Zip:_____

Telephone:_____

Email address:_____

Sales tax: We will add appropriate sales tax for books
shipped to California addresses.

Shipping by air: We will add…
US: $5 for the first book + $2 for each additional book.
International: $10 for the first book + $5 for each add'l book.

Credit card type: [ ] Visa   [ ] MasterCard   [ ] AmEx

Card number:_____

Name on card:_____Exp. Date: ____/____

Signature:_____
* Quantity pricing available upon request